HIV/AIDS and human development in sub-Saharan Africa

AF735134

HIV/AIDS and human development in sub-Saharan Africa

Impact mitigation through agricultural interventions

An overview and annotated bibliography

AWLAE SERIES No. 3

Tanja R. Müller

Wageningen University

Wageningen Academic Publishers

Subject headings:
HIV/AIDS
Human development
Impact mitigation

Foto cover:
Stefan Boness – IPON

ISBN 9076998507
ISSN 1574-2474

First published, 2005

Wageningen Academic Publishers
The Netherlands, 2005

All rights reserved.
Nothing from this publication may be reproduced, stored in a computerised system or published in any form or in any manner, including electronic, mechanical, reprographic or photographic, without prior written permission from the publisher, Wageningen Academic Publishers, P.O. Box 220, NL-6700 AE Wageningen, The Netherlands.

The individual contributions in this publication and any liabilities arising from them remain the responsibility of the authors.

The publisher is not responsible for possible damages, which could be a result of content derived from this publication.

Abstract

This last part of the AWLAE series on HIV/AIDS and agriculture in sub-Saharan Africa focuses on the epidemic as a challenge to human development in general and rural development in particular. In the face of the impact of the epidemic as described in parts one and two of the series, the agricultural sector can potentially play an important role in mitigating some of its effects. Strategies for agricultural intervention are of particular importance in sub-Saharan Africa, given the fact that most of the countries hardest hit by the epidemic are heavily reliant on agriculture. Different agricultural sector based mitigation strategies are discussed. It is further argued, however, that such interventions need to be complemented by interventions from the health and other sectors, in particular by treatment regimes including access to antiretroviral drugs. The text is followed by an annotated bibliography.

Table of contents

Preface

This publication is the last in a three part series being produced within the context of the AWLAE Project based at Wageningen University and Research Centre (WUR). AWLAE stands for African Women Leaders in Agriculture and the Environment, a pan-African programme based in Nairobi, Kenya, within the Leadership Development Division of Winrock International. The overall objectives of AWLAE are to enhance food security and sustainable natural resource management by improving rural women's access to productive resources and technologies, and to ensure greater participation of women in overall decision making.

The AWLAE Project at Wageningen is a doctoral research and training programme in scientific and leadership skills, carried out in partnership with Winrock, the pan-African AWLAE Steering Committee, and AWLAE Alumni. It is funded by the Dutch Ministry of Foreign Affairs (DGIS). Within its parameters, 20 African women from 11 different countries come to Wageningen for their doctoral degree (PhD) in the period 2002 to 2007. The 11 participating countries cover much of Africa's regional diversity. They include from eastern Africa Uganda, Tanzania, Kenya and Ethiopia; from southern Africa Zimbabwe and South Africa; and from western Africa Nigeria, Ghana, Senegal, Benin and Côte d'Ivoire. The project leader is Dr. Julia Gitobu who is based in the Winrock/AWLAE office in Nairobi as regional director. At WUR, the chair group of Sociology of Consumers and Households manages the project and chairs the Academic Advisory Committee (for more information see the WUR website at http://www.socialsciences.wur.nl/sch).

The overall theme of the AWLAE Project is twofold: the role of women in food systems in rural sub-Saharan Africa on the one hand, combined with the impact of HIV/AIDS on food and livelihood systems on the other. Having said that, however, the actual research topics of the PhD candidates are rather diverse, comprising not only a focus on agricultural knowledge and technologies to increase rural women's capacity for food production, processing and marketing, but equally such issues as the potential role of micro-finance institutions to empower women, questions of access to education for rural girls versus boys, and the role of rural women as care-givers - to name just a few examples. What makes the AWLAE project quite unique are the two cross-cutting themes all research projects have to locate themselves within: an emphasis on women's agency and possibilities for its enhancement, and the impacts of HIV/AIDS within a particular research setting.

The body of knowledge being produced within the different PhD research projects will greatly contribute to a better understanding of how different HIV/AIDS epidemics within and between countries and regions - stretching from eastern and southern Africa to western Africa - impact on diverse rural livelihoods and ultimately regional and national options for rural development. As such, it will bring together Anglophone and Francophone research findings and discourses which to this day often rarely take notice of each other, with the ultimate objective of increased networking and sharing of experiences among women researchers from the various geographical settings.

Additionally, in looking at issues of wider rural development in relation to HIV/AIDS through the lens of implications for women's agency, the project is expected to contribute to more gender conscious policies in the future. Given the gendered nature of agricultural livelihoods, combined with the gendered impacts of HIV/AIDS, female scholars in particular can provide relevant policy analysis. In a further step, technically trained women armed with appropriate PhDs can help to bridge the gap between research and policy change.

This publication is the last in a series of three, with the overall objective of providing a resource base on the most crucial issues to consider when looking at rural development in sub-Saharan Africa in a broad sense at the time of HIV/AIDS. The first publication dealt with the impact of HIV/AIDS on the agricultural sector. The second publication explored the linkages between gender and HIV/AIDS, with a focus on rural women and their role in food security and care giving. This third publication discusses the HIV/AIDS epidemic as a wider development issue, in addition to focusing on agriculture-based mitigation strategies and beyond. All three publications comprise two parts: an essay discussing the major issues and summarizing research carried out to date, followed by an annotated bibliography introducing relevant literature.

Taken together, this publication series is meant to serve the wider academic community as well as development practitioners, the latter including national and multinational bodies as well as non-governmental organisations (NGOs) engaged in development assistance projects. It is intended in particular for PhD students and other researchers who work in settings were HIV/AIDS is a crucial factor in rural development and the welfare of rural households.

Lastly, it is hoped that this series helps to contribute to acknowledging the HIV/AIDS pandemic as at present the major challenge to human development in sub-Saharan Africa and beyond. At the same time - in accordance with the objectives of the AWLAE Project - it is meant to give renewed impetus to the need to strengthen women's agency if the promises of human development are to be achieved and the fight against the epidemic is to be won eventually.

Anke Niehof,
Chair AWLAE Academic Advisory Committee
Sociology of Consumers and Households Group (SCH) - WUR

Acknowledgement: The author wishes to acknowledge the financial support from the Dutch Ministry of Foreign Affairs (DGIS) that made the research for this book possible.

List of acronyms

ACT	African Conservation Tillage Network
AESA	Agro-Economic Systems Analysis
AIDS (SIDA)	Acquired Immune Deficiency Syndrome
ANRS	Agence Nationale de Recherches sur le SIDA
ART	Anti-Retroviral Therapy
ARVs	Anti-Retroviral Drugs
AWLAE	African Women Leaders in Agriculture and the Environment
BBC	British Broadcasting Corporation
DFID	UK Department for International Development
DGIS	Dutch Ministry of Foreign Affairs
DIIS	Danish Institute for International Studies
DOT	Directly-Observed Therapy
EQUINET	Regional Network for Equity in Health in Southern Africa
FANTA	Food and Nutrition Assistance Project
FAO	United Nations Food and Agricultural Organisation
FFS	Farmer Field School
FLS	Farmer Life School
GDP	Gross Domestic Product
GTZ	Deutsche Gesellschaft für Technische Zusammenarbeit
HAART	Highly Active Anti-Retroviral Treatment
HDI	Human Development Index
HEARD	Health Economics and HIV/AIDS Research Division, University of Natal
HESA	Human Eco-System Analysis
HIV (VIH)	Human Immunodeficiency Virus
HPI	Human Poverty Index
HSRC	Human Sciences Research Council, South Africa
IAEN	International AIDS Economics Network
IAVI	International AIDS Vaccine Initiative
IDS	Institute of Development Studies Brighton
IFAD	International Fund for Agricultural Development
IFPRI	International Food Policy Research Institute

iied	International Institute for Environment and Development
IMAGE	Intervention with Microfinance for AIDS and Gender Equity
IMF	International Monetary Fund
IOM	International Organisation for Migration
LSTs	Labour Saving Technologies
MDGs	Millennium Development Goals
NEPAD	New Partnership for Africa's Development
NGO	Non-Governmental Organisation
ODI	Overseas Development Institute London
PhD	Doctor of Philosophy
PLWHA	People Living With HIV/AIDS
PPP	Purchasing Power Parity
PVO	Private Voluntary Organisation
RENEWAL	Regional Network on HIV/AIDS, Rural Livelihoods and Food Security in sub-Saharan Africa
RTCC	Reduced Tillage and Cover Crops
SAPs	Structural Adjustment Programmes
STIs	Sexually Transmitted Infections
TAC	Treatment Action Campaign
TRIPS	Trade-Related Aspects of Intellectual Property Rights
UN	United Nations
UNAIDS	Joint United Nations Programme on HIV/AIDS
UNDP	United Nations Development Programme
UNRISD	United Nations Research Institute for Social Development
USAID	United States Agency for International Development
WB	World Bank
WHO	World Health Organisation
WTO	World Trade Organisation
WUR	Wageningen University and Research Centre

Key concepts

Coping: to overcome a difficult situation in terms of a disaster suffered by an individual, a household or a community; implies that assets are recovered, food production is restored, and the former living standard is regained

Mitigation: to lessen the impact of HIV/AIDS on afflicted or affected individuals, households or communities; acknowledges the fact that after having suffered a disaster people's or communities' capabilities might be severely curtailed, their entitlements in jeopardy and their choices frustrated; mitigation is thus an evolving answer to a difficult situation, based on trying to develop the best possible course of action under severe conditions, without suggesting that this course of action might be a sustainable coping strategy in the longer term; the more successful mitigation strategies allow longer term sustainability and better livelihood outcomes, but short term mitigation strategies can be equally important

HIV/AIDS related concepts

Susceptibility: a) the likelihood of an individual becoming infected with the HIV virus

b) the likelihood of the spread of HIV infection within a country, a population group, an institution, an enterprise, or at household level, as determined by the interaction of a variety of societal attributes

Vulnerability: the likelihood of significant physical, social or economic impact occurring at individual, household, community, institutional or societal level

Incidence: number of new occurrences (infections) in a specified period of time, usually one calendar year

Prevalence: pool of all infections at a given point in time; in the case of HIV/AIDS commonly measured as rate of infection among adult men and women aged 15 to 49 years

Resistance: ability of an individual to avoid infection; or characteristic of a community which due to economic or social parameters is less prone to have a high number of HIV infected people

Resilience: active response of infected persons that enables them to avoid the worst impacts of AIDS at different levels, or to recover to a level accepted as normal; or response of a community to avoid the worst impact and mitigate successfully

Part 1 - Overview

"I am convinced beyond unreasonable doubt that HIV/AIDS is a symptom, just like conflicts and deepening poverty, of 'development gone wrong' in Africa. [...] HIV is saying to those of us who are interested in the development of the [African] continent that it cannot be business as usual. The old, conventional, traditional approaches to development have failed to lift us out of the present crisis. If we cannot think of alternatives, let us at least dialogue. Is HIV a symptom of development gone wrong? If the answer is yes then we need to tackle the disease 'development' as we deal with the symptom 'HIV'."
Dr. Roland Msiska, one-time Project Director of the UNDP Regional Project on HIV and Development in sub-Saharan Africa in a speech in July 1999 (quoted from Barnett & Whiteside, 1999a:17).

"The sole policy intervention that can strengthen resilience and therefore recovery capacity and thus have an immediate and long term effect on food security is provision of anti-retroviral drugs. [...] Above all, antiretroviral treatment will ensure [...] that communities can reproduce themselves socially, economically and nutritionally. This is the path that leads to development and independence rather than dependence and destitution."
Tony Barnett and Rachel Grellier in a consultancy report for DFID on the mitigation of HIV/AIDS impact on rural livelihoods (Barnett & Grellier, 2003:7).

"The challenge presented by HIV/AIDS is a challenge against the established order and its historical legacy, it is a call for intensified struggle to remove exploitation that creates poverty, to provide free medical treatment at point of delivery, to divert resources to the improvement of public health services such as clean water and efficient sewerage, to equalise male and female legal rights and facilitate access to their benefits, to eliminate protectionism by private business interests whether in the form of patent laws or farm subsidies, and to create an effective general education base for both sexes."
Roy Love in the journal Review of African Political Economy (Love, 2004:646-7).

1. Introduction

At the beginning of the twenty-first century, HIV/AIDS poses arguably the most critical development challenge in many countries in sub-Saharan Africa and increasingly beyond.[1]

The HIV/AID pandemic is having a devastating impact on the social and economic development of the countries most severely affected (see for example Loewenson & Whiteside, 1997, for an overview of these issues in the context of southern Africa). It has thus been argued that to speak about 'AIDS-impact' might no longer be appropriate in parts of the African continent, but that 'endemic AIDS' should be the point of departure (Barnett, 2004).

Until quite recently, the predominant understanding of 'AIDS in Africa' has been based on biomedical models of individual risk and rational behavioural change (Kalipeni et al., 2004). In line with such an understanding, the response to HIV/AIDS has focused largely on two areas: firstly, containment of the epidemic in terms of preventing new infections through advocacy, education, information and condom distribution campaigns, and, secondly and rather more slowly, providing care and treatment for people living with HIV/AIDS (PLWHA). Such often politically motivated policy responses have tended to ignore the 'bigger picture' in terms of the dynamics behind the thriving of the pandemic as well as its implications for human development in general and poverty reduction in particular (Loewenson

[1] By the end of 2004, an estimated 39.4 million people worldwide were living with HIV/AIDS. Of these, 25.4 million were living in sub-Saharan Africa, where in 2004 alone an estimated 3.1 million people became newly infected with the human immunodeficiency virus (HIV), while 2.3 million people died of Acquired Immune Deficiency Syndrome (AIDS) (all data from UNAIDS/WHO, 2004). While sub-Saharan Africa remains the region most seriously affected by the epidemic - albeit showing considerable differences within and between countries - emerging epidemics elsewhere, including in the Caribbean, parts of Latin America and Asia, and most notably localised epidemics in India and China, as well as Eastern Europe, parts of which experience some of the fastest growing epidemics in the world, leave little room for complacency (see Barnett, 2003; Stillwaggon, 2000; The Economist, 17 April 2004; UNAIDS, 2004; UNDP, 2004; Zhang, 2004). See also Piot (2005) on the 'exceptionality' of the AIDS pandemic due to the fact that no 'epidemic equilibrium' or 'plateau' is in sight in the foreseeable future.

& Whiteside, 2001; see also Klouda, 1995, on the imposition of political priorities with a simultaneous disregard for the underlying inequalities that lead to poor health or development).

Already, development gains made 'pre-AIDS' in those parts of sub-Saharan Africa where AIDS has become endemic as measured by the Human Development Index (HDI), have been reversed. The HDI is a composite measure based on three basic dimensions of well-being: longevity, measured as life expectancy at birth; educational attainment, measured as the weighted average of adult literacy and gross enrolment ratios; and standard of living, measured as Purchasing Power Parity (PPP) of income equivalent in US dollars (see UNDP, 1990). In most of the in income-terms poor countries of sub-Saharan Africa, advances in the HDI have been related to an increase in life expectancy at birth, coupled with a decrease in infant mortality rates, and it is here that the biggest reversal has occurred.[2] One might argue that life expectancy is too crude an indicator for human development, in itself a highly contentious concept. The understanding of human development underlying this publication is drawn from Amartya Sen, one of the intellectual fathers of the HDI: He defines human

[2] While figures on life expectancy at birth differ, sometimes considerably, between different sources, most notably between UN estimates and estimates by the US Census Bureau (for a detailed discussion see Stover, 1998) both sources show a considerable impact of HIV/AIDS on average life expectancy. One of the most vivid examples of a decline in life expectancy and its connection with HIV/AIDS comes to the fore when comparing Uganda and Botswana. The latter enjoyed a life expectancy at birth almost comparable to rich countries at the outset of the epidemic (66.82 years in 1990). By 2003 Botswana had become one of the countries with the highest HIV prevalence rate, 37.3 percent of the adult population (www.unaids.org, accessed 14 January 2005). In parallel, life expectancy at birth in Botswana had fallen to 38.7 years by 2000, and is projected to fall to 34.6 years in 2025. In contrast, in Uganda, where nationwide HIV prevalence figures have been on the decline from a peak of around 15 percent in 1992 to 4.3 percent in 2003 (Allen & Heald, 2004; Schoepf, 2003) life expectancy at birth stood at 43.44 years in 1990, markedly below that of Botswana. In 2000, however, Uganda's life expectancy at birth was 45.4 years, and is projected to be 62.8 years in 2025 (all data on life expectancy from US Census Bureau, September 2004 release, accessed 14 January 2005). See also Ngom & Clark (2003) for a general discussion of the strong association between the (gendered) probability of premature death and adult HIV prevalence; and de Waal (2003) on adult life expectancy (in contrast to life expectancy at birth) as a particularly useful indicator for understanding socio-economic impacts of the pandemic, as adult expectations of longevity influence decision making in areas such as saving patterns, career choices, and participating in behaviour associated with the risk of HIV transmission.

development in its broadest sense as the expansion of people's 'capabilities' to "lead the kind of lives they value and have reason to value" (Sen, 1999:18).[3] Undoubtedly, and regardless of the 'level of development', not to die prematurely is an important component of such a life, as is to be able to prevent one's children from dying at a young age or before oneself - both happening frequently in high HIV/AIDS prevalence countries.[4]

Moreover, the HIV/AIDS pandemic is bound to prove to be the single biggest obstacle in reaching the so-called Millennium Development Goals (MDGs), agreed on at the United Nations Millennium summit in 2000 with the overall objective to cut world poverty by half by the year 2015 (UN General Assembly, 2000; UN, 2004).[5] In fact, when

[3] This definition encompasses not only the notion of well-being, but more broadly the agency potential of people (for further discussion see Sen, 1993). People's agency potential - or their 'capabilities' - can be enhanced or hindered by public policy. At the same time the direction of public policy can be influenced by "effective use of participatory capabilities by the public" (Sen, 1999:18). This is an important aspect in relation to public policy responses to HIV/AIDS. In settings where the epidemic has been contained, enlightened public policy has played an important part (see Boone & Batsell, 2001; Müller, 2005b; Putzel, 2003; 2004). In other settings, public policy was forced to act by strong civil society action - see for example the role played by the Treatment Action Campaign (TAC) in changing government policy in South Africa (Armstrong, 2003; Robins & von Lieres, 2004; Willan, 2004). While the TAC has relied on ways of mobilisation that have been described as 'globalisation from below' and successfully followed a policy of 'strategic engagement' with the South African state (Robins & von Lieres, 2004), a note of caution seems in order here in that civil associations and NGOs are not necessarily catalysts of civic action and agents of reform (for a more detailed discussion see Boone & Batsell, 2001).

[4] A 'short life', measured as the probability at birth of not surviving to the age of 40, is regarded as one of the most basic indicators of deprivation in the quality of life as measured by the UNDP's Human Poverty Index (HPI) - the other two indicators are a lack of basic education, and a lack of access to public and private resources that allow a 'decent' standard of living (UNDP, 1997). Concerning children's mortality and HIV/AIDS, in the highest HIV prevalence countries in sub-Saharan Africa, namely Swaziland (38.8 percent), Botswana (37.3 percent), Lesotho (28.9 percent) and Zimbabwe (24.6 percent), infant mortality and under five mortality rates have (with the exception of Lesotho where those rates were extraordinarily high in the first place) increased between 1980 and 2001, presumably (partly) because many of the children of infected parents do not survive for very long (mortality data from the World Bank, World Development Indicators 2003; HIV/AIDS prevalence figures from www.unaids.org, accessed 14 January 2005).

[5] For a critique of the general philosophy behind the MDGs as being based not on meaningful redistribution mechanisms but on advocating the neoliberal model of development see Thomas (2000).

looking at the MDGs and other development and poverty reduction targets, they have often been formulated without "taking into account the added challenges resulting from sharp increases in AIDS-related adult mortality rates" (Loewenson & Whiteside, 2001:3; but see Björkman, 2002, on the impossibility to achieve the MDGs or nationally determined poverty targets without an effective response to the AIDS crisis).[6]

Crucial to any effort to combat the pandemic and turn its developmental impact around will thus be a more profound understanding of the linkages between HIV/AIDS and poverty, as well as those between poverty and HIV/AIDS, coupled with the political will to act upon such an understanding. Poverty is defined here as a multidimensional, relational concept. This notion of poverty acknowledges the composite inter-related aspects of well-being that determine a person's quality of life (May, 2001; Msiska, 2002; for a detailed evaluation of different types of poverty assessments see Hanmer et al., 1999). These include material aspects (for example food, income, housing, clothing and so forth) as well as non-material aspects (for example decision making power, social support networks and happiness). Recognition of the relational nature of poverty makes it impossible to arrive at an absolute, universally applicable definition (Msiska, 2002). Instead, poverty needs to be related to the specific life situations of a country's or community's population (May, 2001). In a similar tradition of thinking, poverty has been described as the "*inability* of individuals, households or entire communities to *command* sufficient resources to satisfy a socially acceptable minimum standard of living" (Committee of Inquiry into a Comprehensive System of Social Security for South Africa, 2002:15,

[6] HIV/AIDS does feature in goal number six, which aims to 'combat HIV/AIDS, malaria and other diseases'. The concrete target in terms of combating HIV/AIDS reads as follows: 'Have halted by 2015 and begun to reverse the spread of HIV/AIDS' (Sachs, 2005). What is missing here is an acknowledgement that HIV prevention and AIDS mitigation might additionally need to be addressed within many if not all of the other development goals (Whiteside, 2002). Similarly, Africa's major contemporary development initiative, the New Partnership for Africa's Development (NEPAD), includes - apart from some reference to HIV/AIDS as a public health problem - no consideration of its developmental impact (de Waal, 2003).

my emphasis).[7] It is argued here that it is this - what could be called 'poverty of opportunities' - that should be at the centre of public policy, as it turns the focus on the underlying causes of poverty and allows poverty to be addressed in all its dimensions, not in terms of income or material assets alone, potentially leading to strategies that enhance opportunities. In the face of the HIV/AIDS pandemic, such holistic interventions are called for more than ever - in particular in light of the fact that the relationship between HIV/AIDS and development as well as between the pandemic and poverty is cyclical (Msiska, 2002; see also the discussion on gender and HIV/AIDS in Müller, 2005a). On the one hand, AIDS related morbidity and mortality undermines the capacity and capabilities of individuals, households, communities, individual sectors and the state to pursue development and poverty eradication efforts. On the other hand, the level of development and poverty potentially accelerates or inhibits the progression of the epidemic in a given household or community. Poverty here cannot simply be considered as one co-factor facilitating the spread of the epidemic - alongside biological factors, gender inequalities or cultural dimensions; in contrast, those three factors are often aggravated by poverty (Collins & Rau, 2000; Farmer, 1996).[8]

The different potential and observed pathways of the relationship between HIV/AIDS, development and by implication poverty have been documented at various levels, ranging from the individual to the household, public and private enterprises, and the macro-economy (see Bell et al., 2003 and 2004, Bloom & Mahal, 1997, Brown, 2004, Cuddington, 1993, Cuddington & Hancock, 1995, and Over, 1992, on

[7] Looking in this context at community poverty, this has been described to include - next to a lack of services and infrastructure - instability and disunity, or what could be called a lack of social cohesion (May, 2001). The degree of social cohesion within a society or community has in turn been proposed as an important determinant for the severity of its HIV/AIDS epidemic, with less cohesive societies experiencing larger epidemics (Barnett & Whiteside, 1999b; Müller, 2005b) - the conclusion will come back to this point.

[8] Farmer (1996) argues in this context that it is not gender alone that defines the greater susceptibility of women, but gender constraints intensified by poverty. Poor women are the ones most likely to engage in transactional sexual encounters that carry a high risk of infection (see also Bryceson et al., 2004; Hallman, 2004). Looking at this observation in terms of mitigation strategies, it might be easier, at least in the shorter term, to alleviate poverty (and with it reduce women's susceptibility and vulnerability) than to change deep-seated traditional gender roles.

often contradictory predictions of macro-economic implications and challenges of measurement; de Waal, 2003, on a critical discussion of those pathways within a wider focus on governance; Bollinger et al., 1999, on Tanzania; Bollinger et al., 2000, on Malawi; Booysen, 2003, on South Africa; Price-Smith & Daly, 2004, on Zimbabwe; Müller, 2004a on the agricultural sector; Bennell et al., 2002, World Bank, 2002, and Worst & Arndt, 2004 on the education sector and human capital accumulation).

The relationship between poverty and HIV/AIDS is altogether more difficult to grasp, as there is not much in the way of conclusive research. Having said that, a number of direct or indirect relationships between poverty and the likelihood of HIV transmission and AIDS impact have been documented.[9] Poverty, often coupled with food insecurity, may drive women into transactional sexual encounters that carry a high risk of HIV transmission (see Müller, 2005a for a more general discussion; Gillespie et al., 2001 on relations with food and nutrition security; Bryceson et al., 2004 and Shah et al., 2002 on concrete examples from Malawi).[10]

[9] It has to be pointed out here that the relationship between poverty and HIV/AIDS is not simplistic. While the majority of PLWHA in sub-Saharan Africa are poor, and poor people infected with HIV are considerably more likely to develop AIDS as they are likely to be more malnourished, and to lack health attention and medication (see Collins & Rau, 2000, for more details), many non-poor are also infected or affected. In some parts of sub-Saharan Africa it has for example been shown that initially the better-off, mostly men who could afford to spend money on alcohol and multiple partners, were more likely to be infected (see Bryceson et al., 2004). More broadly, a publication based on data from the late 1980s and early 1990s argues that in the first decades of the HIV/AIDS epidemic in sub-Saharan Africa, there was a positive correlation between HIV infection and socio-economic status as measured by income, schooling or occupation - thus disputing the expectation, based on observed higher infection rates with Sexually Transmitted Infections (STIs) among the poor, that poverty, often coupled with illiteracy, raises the probability of HIV infection. But the study argues further that, as HIV/AIDS has become an endemic disease in many African countries, a shift in the pattern of infection to those with lower socioeconomic status has indeed got under way (for a detailed discussion of those findings see Ainsworth & Semali, 1998; in addition see the discussion in Glynn et al., 2004; Gregson et al., 2001; Hallman, 2004).

[10] One needs to be aware in this context of the difference between prostitution and transactional (survival) sex: While prostitutes have a vested interest in protecting their trade and lives and thus in safe sexual encounters, and may have the bargaining power over their clients to enforce safe behaviour, women engaged in transactional sex have neither: It is often rather by chance than planning that they see themselves engaged in such encounters, and they are ill prepared to bargain the terms on which these encounters are taking place (Bryceson et al., 2004; Campbell, 2003).

Poverty often leads to poor diets, which increase susceptibility to HIV infection and hasten the occurrence and progression of opportunistic diseases once a person is infected. Evidence from sub-Saharan Africa has shown that HIV transmission is highly correlated with malnutrition (Stillwaggon, 2000).[11] Poverty increases the likelihood of migration, which in turn may increase a household's or individual's susceptibility to infection (for a discussion of poverty-driven labour migration and the potential social impact of such migration on rural areas see Collins & Rau, 2000).

Furthermore it has been demonstrated that - in addition to gender inequality measured as the gap between adult male and female literacy - both, low income and unequal distribution of income, indicators for an 'uneven form of development', are strongly associated with high HIV infection rates (Gregson et al., 2001; Hallman, 2004; Over, 1998). Such findings lead to the conclusion that economic and social development, "implemented so as to reduce, rather than to increase, income and gender inequality" (Over, 1998:49) is a promising path towards control of the spread of HIV and the mitigation of AIDS impact. Because HIV/AIDS has become part of many poor people's lives, its mitigation will have to include an assault on poverty and its effects on general health (Stillwaggon, 2000). At the same time, policies aimed at poverty alleviation can be crucial to sustain the livelihoods of AIDS afflicted and affected households (Booysen, 2003).

Taken together, the HIV/AIDS pandemic represents a development crisis that deepens poverty and often increases inequality from the

[11] Malnutrition, through its effect on the proper functioning of the immune system, increases susceptibility to STIs in general and HIV in particular (Egal & Valstar, 1999; Stillwaggon, 2000; see also the discussion in Gillespie & Kadiyala, 2005). It is also no coincidence that sub-Saharan Africa, the region most severely affected by the HIV/AIDS pandemic, has the highest percentage of people experiencing food insecurity - in 2002, more than 30 percent of the population of sub-Saharan Africa as a whole was 'undernourished' (see FAO, 2004, also for more country- and region-specific data).

household to the global level (Barnett & Whiteside, 2002).[12] It has social roots and needs a social response, in addition to a technical and medical one. It will be crucial in the future to address the economic, social, political and cultural factors that render individuals and communities susceptible and vulnerable to HIV/AIDS (Kalipeni et al., 2004; Msiska, 2002; Parker et al., 2000). More generally, people's capacity to deal with and respond to the threat of disease is fundamentally shaped by the social and economic conditions they live in, which form their 'vulnerability context'.

This publication is focusing on those conditions in relation to rural and small-scale agriculture-based livelihoods and discusses potential mitigation strategies to transform the vulnerability context in order to counteract the developmental impact of the epidemic.[13] Mitigation has overall been poorly documented, which is not to suggest that there is not a multitude of mitigation responses, but that they have as yet not been systematically recorded (Barnett & Whiteside, 2002; but see USAID, 2003; White, 2002; White & Morton, 2005; as well as the documentation on the website of the Southern African Regional Poverty

[12] It has to be pointed out here that estimates of the scope of the epidemic in different geographical settings often rely on (in a strictly scientific sense) unreliable data and 'proxy' indicators, thus need to be treated with caution. The only two systematically sampled, national population-based surveys of HIV sero-status known to the author within sub-Saharan Africa took place in South Africa in 2002 (see Pettifor et al., 2004, focusing exclusively on Youth aged 15-24; Shisana & Simbayi, 2002, focusing on all age groups) - such surveys are unlikely to be repeated on a wider scale due to the difficulty in conducting them as well as the cost involved. At the same time, this dearth of data does not relieve political leaders from the moral imperative to act on the information available (Whiteside et al., 2003).

[13] Pastoralist livelihoods are not discussed here as the AWLAE projects all focus on 'settled' rural livelihoods. In addition, little is known at present about the workings of HIV/AIDS in pastoralist settings and transhumance (but see Gerald, 2004; Morton, 2003; Roth et al., 1999). This lack of 'knowledge' partially extends to forestry and fishery-based livelihoods (but for the latter see Kipp et al., 1995; Hemrich & Schneider, 1997; Tanzarn & Bishop-Sambrook, 2003; and Allison & Seeley, 2004, for an excellent overview of the wider dynamics between HIV/AIDS and fishing communities, including potential mitigation strategies; in addition, the website of the Sustainable Fisheries Livelihoods Programme, a partnership between DFID, FAO and 25 West-African countries at http://www.sflp.org, accessed 22 February 2005). While pastoralist, forestry-based and fishery-based livelihoods show considerable differences between themselves and in relation to settled smallholder farming, some of the underlying dynamics brought about by the HIV/AIDS pandemic are quite comparable in each setting - they mainly lead to different manifestations.

Network (SARPN) at http://www.sarpn.org.za, accessed 18 April 2005, for an attempt to overcome this deficit). Mitigation as used here is different from coping, which has - rightly so the author believes - been critized on a number of accounts (see Rugalema, 2000, for a detailed discussion). Coping is defined as to overcome a difficult situation in terms of a disaster suffered by an individual, a household, or a community and implies that the former living standard is regained or even surpassed. Looking at an AIDS afflicted household, this implies that such a household can recover assets disposed of, restore food production and so forth (Rugalema, 2000). In contrast to coping, mitigation acknowledges the fact that people's capabilities might be severely curtailed, their entitlements in jeopardy and their choices frustrated. Mitigation is regarded as an evolving answer to a difficult situation, based on an attempt to develop the best possible course of action under severe conditions, without suggesting that this course of action might be a sustainable coping strategy in the longer term. The more successful mitigation strategies allow longer term sustainability and better livelihood outcomes, but short term mitigation strategies can be equally important, might they only consist of community-based organisations that allow AIDS patients to die with dignity. Looking at the 'long wave' nature of HIV/AIDS, manifest in the three stages of the 'HIV/AIDS cycle' - infection and transmission, AIDS induced morbidity and death, and the aftermath of death (Barnett & Whiteside, 1999a; Bryceson et al., 2004) - mitigation strategies are of prime importance in stages two and three, the stages where vulnerability to the impact of the epidemic is already felt. If they prove successful, they will, however, influence prevention of infection and transmission and thus help to prevent the 'cycle' from starting.

Turning to the agricultural sector, it has been argued that policies and programmes that can effectively reduce rural poverty are one of the most efficient ways to help people and communities mitigate the impact of the epidemic and in the long term become more resistant to infection - an objective to be achieved by generating broad-based growth of agricultural income combined with employment opportunities in rural areas (Collins & Rau, 2000; Jayne et al., 2004).[14]

This assertion is disputed by others who argue that poverty is often prevalent in rural areas because "economic and social dynamism is at a low ebb in those areas, and is unlikely to improve under any feasible scenario of intervention" (Ellis & Harris, 2004:ii). Ellis and Harris (2004) further argue that it is in fact livelihood diversification, with mobility as one of the main means, which contributes to positive processes of economic and social change in terms of rural poverty alleviation (see also Reardon, 1997, on household income diversification and rural non-farm labour markets). Caution is urged with regard to the resurgence in interest in agricultural technology as a contributor to poverty reduction in rural sub-Saharan Africa (Ellis & Harris, 2004), a resurgence that seems to have gained momentum with the wider acknowledgement that HIV/AIDS is more than a health issue (see for example FAO, 2003). This acknowledgement might in fact have increased an already present bias against mobility because the latter, be it permanent, temporal or circular, is widely believed to accelerate the spread of the epidemic. What is overlooked within this discourse is that it is not mobility per se, but the conditions under which it occurs that make people susceptible to infection. Or, to put it differently, mobility is a contextual factor that might facilitate, but does not cause the spread of HIV (Bryceson et al. 2004; IOM, 2003). And, taking up an argument advanced by Ellis & Harris (2004), a potentially big difference in alleviating poverty could be made by ending the social exclusion of populations living in informal settlements and urban slums and improving the political and social environment of mobile populations in general (see also IOM, 2003; Sachs, 2005). Such

[14] This argument is based on convictions about rural-led growth strategies dating back to the 1970s, stating that in developing countries economic growth and poverty reduction are best achieved by investing in technological change in particular in small-scale agriculture which provides the means of living to the vast majority of the poor (see Mellor, 1976; Lipton, 1977; Johnston & Kilby, 1975). For a recent investigation into these issues in the context of Latin America see de Ferranti et al. (2005). A similar approach underpins the recently published plan on how to achieve the MDGs where it is stated that "almost every successful development experience has been based on a Green Revolution [or agricultural revolution] at an early stage" (Sachs, 2005:33 and ibid.:68) and development strategies based on progress in agriculture are advocated - albeit combined with a focus on strengthening economic linkages between rural and urban areas (ibid.:); see also the discussion in Commission for Africa (2005).

improvements - in ameliorating the vulnerability context of mobile populations - are in turn bound to alter HIV infection rates among such populations.[15]

Whatever one's own convictions on those issues of rural development and poverty alleviation,[16] what the above debate brings to the fore is that many problems arising from the HIV/AIDS epidemic are not HIV/AIDS specific, but show a larger malaise in development opportunities. Policy responses thus need to address the root causes of wider challenges to human development, they need to have a developmental rather than a HIV/AIDS-specific focus (Topouzis, 1998). Or, to look at it from the other side, rural development policies and programmes in support of in particular poverty alleviation, more food and livelihood security and the 'empowerment' of rural women - all of which are central to the AWLAE project - are at the same time HIV/AIDS prevention and mitigation measures.

The following will thus look in more detail at potential agriculture-based mitigation policies and strategies. If such mitigation is successful in helping to prolong the lives of AIDS afflicted people and secure their livelihoods, while at the same time giving them and their communities a sense of hope for the future again, they might come to act as preventive tools, much more so than any behavioural change campaign.

---

[15] For a discussion more generally of so-called 'susceptibility and vulnerability pathways' as a tool to demonstrate that the HIV/AIDS journey is not inevitable but that there are lifestyle choices, even within contexts of poverty, that enable people to remain outside the loop of infection and vulnerability, see Bishop-Sambrook (2003a).

[16] In general it is argued here that in today's globalised world in which people are aware of their relative poverty more than ever before in history, and especially young people are prone to develop visions of a future away from agriculture-based livelihoods, to try to restrict their mobility will be - if not unethical - largely futile (as witnessed by the ever increasing numbers of in particular young male 'illegal economic migrants' to the developed world, as well as by the increase in urbanisation rates within the developing world). In addition, within a global economy dominated by rich nations whose agricultural policies prevent developing countries' products to compete on a level playing field, any hope of younger generations that they might improve their material well-being from agricultural activities is further being eroded (see also Love, 2004). Having said that, however, if the case can be made that agricultural activities can be viable and profitable, such livelihoods may become attractive again to pursue. For an excellent discussion of all the issues around rural poverty reduction see Bahiigwa et al. (2004) where the example of Uganda - widely regarded as a 'success' story - is evaluated.

2. HIV/AIDS and development in sub-Saharan Africa: the rationale behind agricultural mitigation strategies

When looking at HIV/AIDS and development in sub-Saharan Africa in general, and at potential mitigation strategies outside the health sector in particular, the latter need to be envisaged more broadly than with regard to the agricultural sector only.[17] Here the focus will, however, rest with smallholder agricultural and rural livelihoods, for the following reasons: Over two thirds of the population is said to be rural in many sub-Saharan African countries, and there are reasons to believe that the absolute number of PLWHA is higher in rural than in urban areas (du Guerny, 2002a; Topouzis, 1998; see also the discussion in Müller, 2004a).[18] Most of those afflicted or affected by the epidemic in rural areas owe big parts of their livelihood security to (smallholder) agricultural activities (Topouzis & du Guerny, 1999). In addition, poverty assessments for the whole of sub-Saharan Africa typically find poor people overwhelmingly residing in rural areas and

[17] Just to give one example: It has been argued that subsidizing school uniforms and school fees for adolescent girls might do more to reduce HIV transmission than any peer education programme, as it eliminates much of the need for 'sugar daddies'. It is at the same time bound to reduce unwanted pregnancy, raise the age of marriage and over the longer term promote gender equality (Heise & Elias, 1995).

[18] Note should be taken here of the fact that this distinction between rural and urban is often misleading and fails to take into account the complexity of interdependences between the two sectors (see Ellis & Harris, 2004; Ellis, 2000; and James, 2001, on the intimate interdependence between rural and urban as sources not only of income but also of identity; see also Shisana & Simbayi (2002), where it was found that HIV prevalence in South Africa is highest in 'informal urban settlements'; the same is true for 15-24 year old South Africans only, see Pettifor et al., 2004). Zulu et al. (2004), in a study based on data from slum settlements in Nairobi, argue that populations in such settlements are becoming increasingly disadvantaged compared to their rural counterparts in terms of reproductive health services and other social development indicators. In addition, sub-Saharan Africa is urbanising far more rapidly than developed countries and nearly twice as fast as Asia and Latin America. While in 1998, 28 percent of Africans lived in cities, today this number is estimated to be 37 percent and expected to rise to 50 percent by 2020 (Commission for Africa, 2005). But as the AWLAE programme has its focus specifically on rural livelihoods, those are in the centre of discussion here.

a majority of rural people to be poor (World Bank, 1996).[19] It has indeed been argued that food insecurity - a clear indicator of poverty - at rural household level is one of the major factors increasing such a household's susceptibility to HIV infection, as some of its members (usually women or girls) need to turn to survival sex to secure their basic needs (see for example Bryceson et al., 2004, in relation to Malawi; Loevinsohn & Gillespie, 2003, in relation to southern Africa).

It is thus widely accepted by now that HIV/AIDS affects many aspects of the rural economy in the high prevalence countries of sub-Saharan Africa and will continue to do so.[20] In turn, agriculture is bound to have a special role to play in mitigating the epidemic's impact, and rural development projects can potentially play a catalytic role in reducing vulnerability to AIDS impact and susceptibility to HIV infection in due course (du Guerny, 2002a; FAO, 2003; Jayne et al., 2004; Muelder, 2002; Topouzis & du Guerny, 1999). This is in particular the case as for a majority of high prevalence countries in sub-Saharan Africa predominantly dependent on agriculture it is assumed that agriculture related activities and rural development are the prerequisites for an overall structural transformation process that will eventually lead to human development and poverty eradication (Jayne et al., 2004).[21]

[19] For a critical discussion of the methods used to arrive at poverty figures in World Bank reports see Hanmer et al. (1999). While much of the criticism formulated by Hanmer et al. (1999) is shared by the author, the overall finding that poverty in sub-Saharan Africa is predominately rural in many settings is confirmed by many qualitative studies, not least those discussed in the first part of this series in relation to HIV/AIDS and rural livelihoods (see Müller, 2004a). A particularly graphic example of the connection between HIV/AIDS, poverty and rurality is Malawi. It has the eighth highest HIV/AIDS prevalence worldwide, while it is one of the least urbanised countries within sub-Saharan Africa with 85 percent of the population living in rural areas. At the same time, it is one of Africa's poorest countries (Bryceson et al., 2004).

[20] A survey across fifteen African countries conducted by Afrobarometer found that rural people are more likely to care for sick household members, while more generally people living in poverty are more likely to spend time both looking after orphans and taking care of sick household members (Afrobarometer, April 2004, http://www.afrobarometer.org, accessed 24 February 2005).

[21] Ellis & Harris (2004) question this notion and argue that the least vulnerable segments of the rural population are those least dependent on agriculture (see also Brown et al., 1994). A study from Malawi suggests that while smallholder agricultural growth is vitally important to 'pro-poor' growth in the rural non-farm informal economy, its stimulus is not enough to reduce high rates of poverty if other drivers are missing (Dorward, 2003).

Agricultural interventions can be considered at two levels: the farming system level and the farm-household system level (du Guerny, 2002a; see Müller, 2004a for further discussion of those two levels). The latter is where the majority of HIV/AIDS impact studies has been conducted - even though the particular pathways of such impacts and their magnitude remain by and large unclear (Jayne et al., 2004) - and where mitigation efforts have their focus. One should keep in mind, however, that interventions at the farm-household system level, in particular if they occur on a larger scale, will eventually have repercussions for the farming system level, for the better or worse. At the same time, broader economy-wide developments that occur - either as a result of the epidemic or due to other causes - will have their repercussions for the agricultural system and with those will be felt at the farm-household level.[22]

The precise pathways of HIV/AIDS impact on rural smallholder agricultural livelihoods are far from clear. Research is thus called for to understand with greater precision how the rural socio-economy is being affected in order to be able to modify agricultural and rural development policies in a way that helps better to achieve national agricultural policy objectives while at the same time mitigate HIV/AIDS impact (Jayne et al., 2004). Having said that, however, a general assumption in the literature as well as in popular discussions of such impact is that AIDS-related mortality results first and foremost in severe labour constraints, coupled with increased poverty and land scarcity among afflicted households (Mather et al., 2004b). Concerning agriculture-based mitigation strategies, they have in due course been prioritising technology assistance in the form of agricultural labour-saving technologies to make up for the loss of adult labour, often coupled with food aid targeting to AIDS afflicted households (Mather et al. 2004b; see Kraak et al., 1999 for a discussion of the potential role of food aid in AIDS mitigation). Two other areas that have received attention are to combat the loss of knowledge incurred by the premature death of prime age adults, as well as to address the weaknesses within agricultural extension services. The former is most prominent in the

[22] Jayne et al. (2004), give the example of a macro-economic decline in the form of Gross Domestic Product (GDP) contraction, which is bound to effect demand and price levels for agricultural commodities. At the same time, many of the effects of HIV/AIDS on the agricultural sector are bound to operate through the overall economy (ibid.).

promotion of farmer field schools, often extended to include a life skills component dealing with HIV/AIDS-related issues; the latter has a focus on gearing extension services towards Youth and women farmers to fill a void created by the dominant focus in the past on the male heads of farming households (see Page, 1999).

The following section will discuss some of these proposed and pursued agriculture-based HIV/AIDS mitigation efforts focusing on areas in which the agricultural sector has a 'comparative advantage' (du Guerny, 2002a) in contributing to such efforts. This discussion is based on the following two premises: Firstly, to prove successful in the longer term, agricultural mitigation strategies need to do both, strengthen the resilience of individuals and households, as well as that of the wider community. Secondly, the most successful strategies to incorporate HIV/AIDS into agricultural sector policies are likely to be "multi-pronged approaches that recognize the varied resource constraints affecting AIDS-afflicted households" (Jayne et al., 2004:15). Mainstreaming HIV/AIDS into agricultural policies thus needs to take into account the social and economic factors that make up the context of the pandemic. This implies for example more than the inclusion of prevention messages at meetings between agricultural extension workers and farmers, but rather the training of extension workers to recognize signs of agricultural stress due to labour shortages or asset constraints. It might require not only the promotion of labour-saving technologies or labour-sharing systems, but to encourage better credit facilities for small farmers, or to reintroduce food or fertiliser subsidies - in short, to do better what needs to be done in any case to develop the rural economy (Bonnard, 2002; Collins & Rau, 2000; see also the discussion in Hemrich & Schneider, 1997, on HIV/AIDS and technical cooperation; and the comprehensive discussion on mainstreaming in Holden, 2003).[23]

---

[23] What exactly the appropriate policy options are is dependent on the overall context. It has for example been suggested that in an agricultural country like Kenya there is great potential for developing employment opportunities and keeping labour in the rural areas; special projects could for example be assigned for AIDS orphans and extension services could focus on this group (Ayieko, 1997). Such proposals might not be relevant to other settings (see also the discussion in Hallman, 2004).

3. Agriculture-based mitigation strategies: potential and pitfalls

Since the first studies on the potential and observed impact of HIV/AIDS on agriculture and rural livelihoods, labour shortages due to premature adult morbidity and mortality, both, in terms of the availability and allocation of labour, have been at the centre of debate (see for example Gillespie, 1989; Barnett & Blaikie, 1992; Barnett et al., 1995; for a general discussion of available research see Müller, 2004a; White & Robinson, 2000). The first response of an afflicted farming household has thus been reported to be the adoption of measures to 'downshift' agricultural activities and reallocate labour within the farm-household interface (Barnett & Grellier, 2003). This scenario seems to suggest labour saving technologies (LSTs) as a promising mitigation strategy from the agriculture sector to counter the pandemic's impact on labour (du Guerny, 2002b).

LSTs are understood here in a broad sense as labour saving methods and inputs in agricultural production and at the farm-household labour interface. They may focus on mechanisation; low-input agriculture; improved tools; improved seed varieties; improved use of fertilizer; improved harvesting methods; but also improved access to water or fuel efficient stoves to reduce the burden on domestic labour (Barnett & Grellier, 2003; du Guerny, 2002b).

While it is advocated that a healthy mistrust be kept at the back of the reader's mind towards the "conventional narrative that equates rural poverty reduction with technical efforts to raise yields in agriculture" (Ellis & Harris, 2004:16), a narrative that among other things neglects the macroeconomic local and global context affecting demand and price levels for agricultural commodities (see Jayne et al., 2004), the potential usefulness of such technical efforts deserves a closer look.

Prominent among the LSTs that have been propagated as particularly useful for vulnerable households is conservation agriculture because its principles are regarded particularly relevant to the context created by HIV/AIDS (see Steiner et al., 2004, for a brief introduction). It is therefore used here as the example to discuss promises and pitfalls of LSTs to mitigate the impact of HIV/AIDS on rural smallholder communities more generally.

Broadly speaking, conservation agriculture aims to enhance agricultural production on a sustainable basis in following three principles: minimum soil disturbance or no tillage; maintenance of a permanent soil cover; and diversified crop rotation (Bishop-Sambrook, 2003b). In doing so, it has the potential to reduce time constraints and labour requirements for land preparation and weeding especially in peak seasons; to contribute to household food security in for example making more efficient use of rainwater and increasing soil fertility through the introduction of cover crops; and to increase household income in generating additional revenue through the production of fodder and cash cover crops (see Bishop-Sambrook et al., 2004, for a more extensive discussion).

Looking at the first of those issues, the reduction of time and labour constraints, this is mainly due to less time spent on land preparation and weeding - both tasks generally ranked by women and men as their most onerous agricultural activities (Bishop-Sambrook, 2003b). Weeding in particular is in many cultures regarded as a woman's task, and a number of studies have shown that weeding activities suffer once women fall ill or are called upon in their role of carers for other sick members of the household (see the discussion in Müller 2004a; 2005a). In addition, conservation agriculture practices allow for many agricultural tasks to be spread over greater periods of time, thus reducing labour intensity at peak times, another constraint often found in HIV/AIDS affected communities that leads to a decline in agricultural production (ibid.). And while eventually to apply conservation agricultural techniques comprehensively would lead to the emergence of a new farming system, one can use some of its practices within an existing system or as a way of drawing additional resources into such a system - thus different levels of technological change can be pursued based on the characteristics of each farming community (Bishop-Sambrook, 2003b). All those characteristics on the face of it suggest conservation agriculture as a particular relevant LST in the context of HIV/AIDS.

What is overlooked here, however, is the fact that each technological change has its initial cost. Looking at conservation agriculture, it has been shown that - depending on who is adopting the technology - it may take considerable amounts of time to reap labour saving benefits.[24] In addition, conservation agriculture has substantial start up cost in terms of purchases of inputs before the benefits of improved soil fertility and crop rotation become fully visible. It has in fact been estimated that it will take between two and five years until such benefits can be reaped (Bishop-Sambrook et al., 2004), a time horizon unlikely to be viable among households hit by AIDS induced morbidity or mortality. With regard to this last point, it has been suggested more generally that too little attention is being paid to the fact that HIV/AIDS is making "foreshortening" a more and more common fact for many in sub-Saharan Africa (Richards, 1999, referring in particular to Youth), and that in turn technology "should help us not to sustain, but dodge and weave" (ibid.:8).

This discussion of conservation agriculture as a potential LST to mitigate AIDS-induced labour shortage raises some additional questions concerning the suitability and sustainability of propagating LSTs to mitigate HIV/AIDS impact on smallholder agriculture.

Firstly, already vulnerable households will not have the resources to meet any start-up cost,[25] and apart from being unable are bound to be unwilling to expose their households to additional risks that might further threaten the existence of an already fragile livelihood base (Bishop-Sambrook, 2003b). Available evidence shows that the poorest and most vulnerable households in a community rarely benefit from

[24] The study by Bishop-Sambrook et al. (2004) reports that for a group of widow farmers who for the first time used the jab planter required for conservation agriculture planting activities - although they saved time on land clearance and weeding - total labour increased initially by fifteen percent, as these women were unfamiliar with the technology. In contrast, men who worked as hired agricultural labourers showed great interest in the jab planter and mastered it quickly (ibid.:31).

[25] Such cost come in cash and kind, and such households have neither the spare cash to purchase new inputs nor the time and labour to invest in adopting new strategies (Bishop-Sambrook, 2003b).

new projects (Barnett & Grellier, 2003; but see Bishop-Sambrook et al., 2004, for an example of how poor female-headed households in the study area did indeed do so; and some of the examples reported in White, 2002; and White & Morton, 2005).[26] More generally, vulnerable households will have to rely on external funding if they are to adopt any LSTs, no matter how beneficial those might turn out to be over the longer term. Such external funding is largely provided by outside donors, and here lies one of the major general problems with the introduction of LSTs: Any attempt to introduce often substantial changes to agricultural systems in the course of the promotion of LSTs needs ideally to be accompanied by long-term technical support, coupled with an adequately designed and funded safety net covering the time before the anticipated benefits take hold, whereas donors usually shy away from such long-term commitments (Barnett & Grellier, 2003).[27] This raises another concern: if newly introduced LSTs such as conservation agriculture prove to be unsustainable over the longer-term within a particular environment (or as soon as donor funding is running out), who will bear the cost? Most likely, it will be the already vulnerable who might end up worse off than before - thus a rush to ill considered technical innovation could become an additional cost associated with the impact of the HIV/AIDS epidemic (ibid.).

Secondly, activities in relation to LSTs are highly cultural in their expression, a fact often insufficiently taken into account. While Bishop-Sambrook et al. (2004) for example acknowledge that the adoption of conservation agriculture requires a significant change not only in farming practices but equally "a fundamental change in mindset towards cultivation practices" (ibid.:6), this last component or how to arrive at such a change is not discussed any further in the concluding chapter where the potential of conservation agriculture is evaluated

[26] More generally there is evidence that in any setting the poor are least likely to be among early adopters of new technologies; it are the more wealthy that innovate and adopt more readily, but the latter are also those who cope better with HIV/AIDS in the first place (Barnett & Grellier, 2003). Having said that, however, a number of studies have shown that illiterate and usually poorer neighbours of more educated farmers benefit by simply watching and copying innovations of the latter (see the examples discussed in Worst & Arndt, 2004).

[27] The majority of LST interventions discussed by Barnett & Grellier (2003) for example had funding assured for no more than three years.

based mainly on its 'technical' components.[28] Most of the documented experiences with LSTs to date dichotomise technical and social HIV/AIDS mitigation strategies, resulting in a lack of synthesis between the technical and social aspects of agricultural production and rural livelihoods. Collaboration between technical specialists and social scientists would give much better insights into for example the processes of adoption or rejection of innovation, and increase the exploration of context-appropriate technologies (Barnett & Grellier, 2003).[29] It is in this area that the AWLAE project can make an important contribution, in particular the work of Susana Akrofi, Faith Nguthi and Monica Karuhanga.[30]

Thirdly, the rationale that suggests LSTs as main focus of AIDS mitigation to be pursued by agricultural research and extension systems is put more and more into question (Jayne et al., 2004; Mather et al., 2004b). Advocates of LSTs tend to argue that many smallholder households even without HIV/AIDS already face labour shortages. HIV/AIDS impact does mainly accentuate those shortages and forces households into often irreversible coping strategies (Bishop-Sambrook, 2003b). Many of the technologies advocated for such households to better wither the impact of the epidemic are in fact not new, but are being reintroduced with the expectation of a better take-up, as households are now so desperate that they will grab any chance offering a betterment of their situation. HIV/AIDS is thus acting quasi as the catalyst for potentially more successful LST implementation (see Bishop-Sambrook et al., 2004). Apart from the more general observation

[28] Barnett & Grellier (2003) for example mention as a socio-cultural aspect hindering the adoption of conservation agricultural practices the fact that fields look 'untidy' whilst social pressure to maintain a 'clean' appearance of fields has been observed.

[29] An example of what could be achieved by interventions that not only focus on a concrete and measurable outcome but at the same time pay attention to underlying structural factors driving the epidemic is reported in Kim et al. (2002), albeit not based on LSTs but on microfinance projects targeting poor rural women.

[30] Susana Akrofi's research project is entitled 'Effects of HIV/AIDS Affliction on Management Strategies in Home Gardens in Southern Ghana with Special Reference to Biodiversity', Faith Nguthi is working on 'Suitability of New Agricultural Technologies in HIV/AIDS Affected Farming Households: The Case of the Tissue Culture Banana in Kenya', and Monica Karuhanga on 'An Assessment of the Interrelationships between HIV/AIDS, Intra- and interhousehold Dynamics and Banana Technology Uptake in the Masaka and Kabarole Districts of Uganda.'

that agricultural innovation and its adoption in sub-Saharan Africa during and since the colonial period does not demonstrate that these processes have been either well understood nor proved effective, it has to be doubted that increasing desperation provides an additional incentive for technology uptake (Barnett & Grellier, 2003).

In addition, more recent research demonstrates that AIDS afflicted and affected households do not necessarily have less prime-adult labour available than non-affected households,[31] nor do they necessarily change cultivation patterns or experience effects on crop income - leading to the conclusion that labour does not necessarily become the limiting input in agricultural production (see Beegle, 2003; Mather et al., 2004b).[32] In contrast, gender and household position of the deceased, together with the asset level of a household appear to determine household-level effects (ibid.; see also Yamano & Jayne, 2004; and the discussion in Müller, 2004a). Moreover, in a majority of settings featuring in the study by Mather et al. (2004b) the deceased prime-age adults were not the household heads or spouses,[33] but other, often younger female members of the household - leading to the assumption

[31] This assertion does not consider the potential demographic response by a household in terms of admitting new members. Research from Kagera, Tanzania, has for example indicated that rural households often maintain household size and dependency ratios after experiencing prime-age adult death (see the discussion in Beegle, 2003; see also Mather et al., 2004b).

[32] Looking at the macro-level picture suggests that while the AIDS pandemic will reduce life expectancy and population growth in the hardest-hit countries of sub-Saharan Africa, it will most likely not result in a decline in the aggregate labour-to-available-land ratio (Mather et al., 2004b). More generally, questioning the widely-held assumption - often based on anecdotal evidence from few settings - that agricultural labour is the limiting factor to food security and sustainable livelihoods in the high-prevalence countries of sub-Saharan Africa can be 'politically' sensitive: An informal paper circulated by an organisation working in that field questioning 'all the fuss about agricultural labour and HIV/AIDS' drew an angry response from staff members of one of the leading international organisations working on AIDS and agriculture (personal correspondence with some of the people involved who wish to remain anonymous).

[33] Taking for example the case of Mozambique, survey results there show that only one third of prime-age adults who had died prematurely were household heads or spouses of household heads (Mather et al., 2004a). Contrasting findings have, however, been reported from eastern Zimbabwe: A study by Mushati et al. (2003) found that among surveyed households more than three quarters had lost their predominant income earner to premature death, and deceased persons were more likely to be household heads when the cause of death was HIV-associated.

that the impact of prime-age adult mortality on rural household agricultural and off-farm income may be less than commonly predicted (ibid.).[34] This trend is in line with more general data on the increasing number of HIV infections among younger women in sub-Saharan Africa. The intention here is not to play done the potentially devastating impact of the pandemic on rural communities, but to question the rationale behind many mitigation strategies, in particular those based on LSTs.[35]

Such technologies might indeed be appropriate for certain households and more research here is certainly welcome and needed[36] - and here again the AWLAE programme can provide a valuable contribution. What Mather et al. (2004b) also found is that certain types of households, including poor widow headed households as a prime example (in line with previous research, see the discussion in Müller, 2005a), faced by far the biggest problems. They thus suggest that interventions addressing the gender bias in agricultural production and marketing

[34] The study cited here also found relatively few occurrences of household dissolution in Kenya, Malawi and Rwanda (Mather et al., 2004b). These findings counter some of the critics of survey based data who claim that households with prime-adult death frequently dissolve and are not recorded, resulting in biased data sets (see also Mushati et al., 2003).

[35] The research conducted by AWLAE student Rose Fagbemissi will be concerned with this set of questions. In her research location in Benin, households tend to hire agricultural labour and pay for such labour with income from other activities. When AIDS hits the household, the immediate problem is thus the loss of that income, possibly coupled with inadequate agricultural knowledge. Her concrete research topic is 'Knowledge and Integrated Pest Management Problem-Solving by Orphans and Young Farmers in the Context of HIV/AIDS in Benin'.

[36] Findings from survey-based research in Mozambique indicate for example that 44 percent of households afflicted by premature prime-age mortality reduced crop planting areas, while 22 percent reduced weeding as a coping strategy suggesting that labour constraints are indeed a concern for some households (Mather et al., 2004a). In a similar vein, findings from Rwanda indicate that around 60 percent of households in which a prime adult (here defined as between 15 and 60 years of age) died of illness reduced farm-labour inputs, leading to less land being cultivated - strategies to shift to less labour-intensive crops were, however, not common (Donovan et al., 2003). It should be pointed out here that a reduction in output of subsistence crops, in particular when not accompanied by a similar reduction in other crop output, need not indicate per capita changes in household output: prime adult death not only constitutes a loss of labour, but equally causes a reduction in the number of household members consuming food and other goods (Beegle, 2003).

knowledge, or better land security for widows, could contribute significantly to the opportunities of such households to mitigate HIV/AIDS impact (ibid.; see also Aliber et al., 2004). More widely it has been suggested that interventions should be based on the intention of improving overall livelihood parameters, which is bound to lead to a targeting of widows, orphans and young people among others (see White, 2002). Targeted interventions to mitigate HIV/AIDS impact are often related to a transfer of goods, often in the form of food-aid, or money, the latter often in the form of micro-credit schemes.

The introduction of LSTs is often combined with such targeted interventions or relies on micro-credit schemes to get off the ground. Even though micro-credit schemes are certainly not the silver bullet they are sometimes propagated to be, in particular for resource-poor households they can indeed have a vital function. Research from Kagera district in Tanzania has for example shown that resource-abundant households can and do rely to a large extent on private transfers to mitigate the impact of HIV/AIDS, whereas resource-poor households often have no opportunity to secure such transfers and therefore rely relatively more on credit. It has thus been argued that to the extent to which micro-credit programmes improve access to borrowing and lower its cost they might be an effective tool to help the most resource-poor households to cope with the impact of premature adult mortality due to AIDS (Lundberg, Over & Mujinja, 2000; White, 2002).[37] In addition, evidence from Uganda suggests that even if individual training or credit schemes have been unsuccessful, they might have a longer term effect in that the provision of training combined more generally with capacity building has enabled women's groups to obtain credit from external organisations where their gender, poverty and lack of

[37] The work of two AWLAE students will shed some more light on these issues, Hirut Bekele and Namizata Binate. Hirut Bekele's work is entitled 'Women's Participation in Microfinance Programmes and Changes in Intra-household Gender Division of Labour and Decision Making Power: The Case of Sidama Microfinance Institution in Ethiopia', while Namizata Binate is working on 'The efficacy of micro-financing of women's agricultural and non-agricultural activities in a high-prevalence HIV/AIDS zone in Côte d'Ivoire.'

assets would previously have prevented them from doing so (Barnett & Grellier, 2003).[38]

More generally, in particular group-based microfinance interventions have been demonstrated to foster enhanced autonomy and resilience among women participants, with newly acquired economic and business skills translating into self esteem, improved social networks, and wider control over household decision making processes. Specific research on the health impacts of such schemes has shown improvements in the nutritional intake and educational status of children, and a greater likelihood of contraceptive use among participants as compared to control groups, the latter an important aspect in terms of sexual decision making power (see the discussion in Kim et al., 2002). Having said that, however, the links between microfinance and empowerment are complex. While it has been argued that projects which help to enhance women's access to financial capital can assist women in developing effective income-generating strategies that benefit their entire family (White, 2002), exactly in what way economic empowerment enhances general well-being, status and autonomy in decision making or not is not well understood (Kim et al., 2002).

This leads to the last point discussed here, a methodology considered particularly relevant for the introduction of LSTs and other agriculture-based mitigation strategies in the context of HIV/AIDS: the Farmer Life School (FLS). FLSs promote a holistic development strategy. Farmers are encouraged to examine their overall life context instead of focusing narrowly on an increase in agricultural production, and to define themselves what it means to them in their particular circumstances to have a 'healthy quality of life' (Sokunthea, 2002). The main focus of a FLS lies on creating an enabling environment through training (FAO, 2003). A FLS is thus held in the houses of participating farmers; during the FLS farmers learn how to conduct a so-called

[38] It should be pointed out here, however, that each income generating activity is in fact a small business. To start such a business is difficult in any setting at the best of times, so how successful such endeavours can be in an already unfavourable context like those in most African countries with the additional threat posed by HIV/AIDS needs to be questioned - such endeavours might thus require the simultaneous introduction of emergency support systems (see White, 2002).

'human eco-system analysis' (HESA) - in doing so, one key objective is for farmers to adopt a more long-term horizon. Traditionally, many farmers are accustomed to think in terms of the agricultural calendar and crop cycle within a given year. A FLS aims to instil a longer term perspective among farmers while at the same time giving participants the confidence that they can actually shape that future to different extents, and make it become meaningful to invest in such a future. Such future oriented strategies will then - it is assumed - help in the reduction of behaviour that exposes farmers to HIV infection. FLSs have thus a double objective: On the one hand the promotion of a vision for a meaningful future, while on the other, in following a FLS farmers can access knowledge on how to avoid HIV infection or deal better with HIV/AIDS impact (du Guerny et al., 2002; FAO, 2003; UNDP and FAO, 2004).[39] More generally, adopting a long-term time perspective has been identified as crucial in HIV prevention (see du Guerny, 2002a; Sokunthea, 2002, for a more extensive discussion).

Taken together, FLSs are in line with the approach towards development advocated in this publication and more generally with changes in development practice towards human-centred approaches premised on participation and people's empowerment (Topouzis & du Guerny, 1999).

The FLS has been pioneered in the context of south-east Asia, mainly in Cambodia, where it seems to have proved highly successful (Sokunthea, 2002; Yech, 2003). Some efforts are now under way in parts of eastern and southern Africa based on an extension of FFS.[40] These

[39] The FLS is basically an extension of the Farmer Field School (FFS). Whereas FFSs are based on agro-eco-systems analysis (AESA) with the objective to promote integrated pest management strategies, FLS are based on human eco-system analysis (HESA) and aim to transform farm management practices in a way that reduces for example the HIV vulnerability context - HIV/AIDS is seen as one part of the issues around chronic illnesses that affect farming families (for a more detailed discussion see du Guerny, 2002a; UNDP and FAO, 2004; Yech, 2003).

[40] The crucial difference between FFSs and FLSs is that in FFSs the fields are the central component of the learning process, whereas in FLSs the lives of the farmers are. Methodologically, it is generally believed that FLSs can only be implemented successfully in a context where FFSs have worked considerably well, where people have already experienced to observe and discuss problems together and formulate solutions (see Bredewold, 2004; Okoth, 2002).

mostly take the from of 'holistic farmer field schools' (Okoth et al., 2002), which implies a main focus on agricultural components but the inclusion of other aspects that have a bearing on rural livelihoods such as HIV/AIDS, nutrition, health care and so forth (ibid.). It has been reported that FFSs in eastern Africa have increased the levels of interaction between farmers and between farmers and extension officers, thus transforming extension services from a top-down model to a partnership (ibid.); in addition, HIV/AIDS awareness and knowledge of potential strategies to prevent infection and mitigate impact is said to have increased (ibid.). Many FFSs were originally geared towards men, but recently efforts have been made to involve women in an attempt to promote indigenous knowledge and new agricultural techniques,[41] improve access to resources, and reduce labour requirements for domestic tasks (Barnett & Grellier, 2003) - as well as to include Youth.[42] The latter aim to teach agricultural techniques while at the same time through a cultural programme build up self-esteem among the participants and teach them wider life skills (Bredewold, 2004).

While too little evidence is available from sub-Saharan Africa at this stage to recommend FLSs as an effective HIV/AIDS prevention and mitigation methodology, they look like a promising way forward to arrive at more holistic, development centred mitigation strategies going beyond HIV/AIDS but looking at the 'wider' picture (see also White, 2002; White & Morton, 2005, on advocacy of using participatory methods to design interventions and work with existing local structures; and Page & Nyakanda, 2003, for practical suggestions on how to facilitate community action). And regardless of whether an outcome of FLSs are more efficient agricultural practices or not, they are valuable in

[41] This includes the promotion of traditional crops that have been neglected or under-utilised as well as the promotion of wild food and/or medical plants (see Gari, 2002).

[42] One such project are the FAO sponsored Junior Farmer Field and Life Schools in Manica district in Mozambique, geared toward orphans and vulnerable children aged between 8 and 18 years (see Bredewold, 2004, for further discussion). Observations from a field visit to those schools report that thus far they focus on the well-being of the participating children in combination with teaching them agricultural skills, while HIV/AIDS is not particularly emphasised (ibid.). It is thus not possible at this stage to make any inferences how or if those schools - in potentially providing a future livelihood strategy - might become a valuable part in any HIV/AIDS prevention and mitigation effort.

developing analytical and decision making skills of groups and individuals, enhancing confidence and raising consciousness, as well as in promoting discussion about communal problems (often for the first time) and creating informal networks (Yech, 2003), all contributing to social cohesion, a potentially decisive factor in combating the HIV/AIDS pandemic (as will be argued in the concluding section in more detail).

More generally, it needs to be understood that HIV/AIDS is a factor endogenous to many aspects of rural livelihoods. Policies need thus incorporate the changes that might already have altered the conditions under which development takes place, and the altered base from which households, communities, and potentially whole societies are able to respond (Barnett & Grellier, 2003). What is needed to combat the pandemic in rural settings in sub-Saharan Africa is "a combination of relief and development activities by organisations working to increase food security and rural livelihoods" (Barnett & Grellier, 2003:80).

Relief activities often rely on direct transfers and are in due course - often wrongly - regarded as purely social-welfare oriented interventions. But research has shown that such transfers not only are having an effect in terms of protection of a minimum standard of living, but equally in terms of promoting longer term sustainability of living standards (Devereux, 2002), as the poor are what can be called 'bricoleurs', they 'innovate' through the force of circumstances and with what little resources they have (Barnett & Grellier, 2003; Loevinsohn & Gillespie, 2003).[43]

An example with particular relevance to HIV/AIDS mitigation that demonstrates the need to consider policies aimed at the introduction of social safety nets is the case of nutritional interventions. Looking at poverty reduction in general (without taking HIV/AIDS explicitly into account) it has been shown that nutritional interventions in the form of targeted food transfers can lead to a sustainable reduction in poverty, not least because improvements in nutrition status lead to

[43] Many of the responding strategies to HIV/AIDS show indeed how 'inventive' the poor are, no matter that some of those (like transactional sex or migration) are regarded as immoral or illegal by some. Such judgements in general seem to the author highly questionable (see also Barnett & Grellier, 2003).

higher labour productivity (for a more detailed discussion of those relationships see Devereux, 2002). Looking at the case of HIV/AIDS, such interventions can be of even more relevance, as adequate nutrition is of prime importance to infected people and can prolong their lives, well-being, and capacity to engage in work considerably.[44] Such interventions, often not liked because of their 'welfarist' underpinnings, might in reality be a better way to mitigate HIV/AIDS impact in rural settings than the introduction of new agricultural technologies and methodologies - not least because such interventions tend to target the most vulnerable, including women and Youth, who might more often than not be unable to adopt LSTs in an overall environment where (adult) men control access to land, tools, or credit, and where many interventions may require men's cooperation (Barnett & Grellier, 2003).[45]

[44] One project explicitly dealing with these interconnections is the Food and Nutrition Assistance Project (FANTA) funded by USAID. FANTA supports integrated food security and nutrition programming to improve the health and well-being of women and children. In sub-Saharan Africa FANTA and its partners support for example nutritional care and food security interventions within AIDS relief efforts in Rwanda, Kenya and Zambia (for more information on FANTA see http://www.fantaproject.org, accessed 18 April 2005, where also a number of documents discussing the linkages between nutrition and HIV/AIDS can be found).

[45] A new study into those issues is at present under way investigating 'community-based technology change for livelihood security in response to HIV and AIDS', carried out jointly by Laura Murphy at Tulane University in New Orleans and Paul Harvey at the Overseas Development Institute in London. The study seeks to learn from technology innovations and adaptations among communities responding to HIV and AIDS throughout Africa. Fieldwork is to be conducted in the course of 2005 and results will subsequently be published.

4. The issue of gender in mitigation

When considering HIV/AIDS mitigation in relation to agriculture-based livelihoods in rural sub-Saharan Africa, women and their dependants should clearly be central to any intervention aimed at tackling the social and economic impact of HIV/AIDS. This should be the case not only because in many parts of rural Africa women play a major role in agricultural production and bear the brunt of caring for the sick (see the discussion in Müller, 2004a; 2005a), but also because the most vivid struggles reported repeatedly in rural settings are those related to gender constraints - a prime example being the difficulties of women to gain access to land (White, 2002).

Even without the HIV/AIDS pandemic gender constraints should be a key concern within rural development projects, given the central role that women play as guardians of food security in most of rural sub-Saharan Africa (Topouzis & du Guerny, 1999; see also the more general discussion on women, food security and development in Scanlan, 2004). In reality, however, agricultural extension services have traditionally focused on single crops, often cash crops traditionally grown by men, and have largely failed to consider the wide range of activities in which women are involved to secure household food security (Quisumbing et al., 1998). Lately a need for women extension workers and contact farmers has been recognised in order to include the knowledge of women within the formal extension services (ibid.). Indeed, many projects under way now include a gender component. But this inclusion more often than not tends to be limited to increasing women's participation in project activities, while not addressing potential changes in the gender division of labour or changes in the overall status of women (see the examples discussed from Uganda, Tanzania, Malawi and Zambia in Barnett & Grellier, 2003). More generally, too many women-centred projects focus solely on welfare issues instead of focusing equally on women's roles as agricultural producers and managers, or on empowering practices (Quisumbing et al., 1998). Concerning this last issue it has to be pointed out, however, that evidence from welfare-oriented women-focused projects where women are involved in sharing agricultural or other activities shows that such endeavours provide emotional support and that women get strength from each other - thus being a potential first step towards empowerment (see for example Barnett & Grellier, 2003, in relation to a project in Malawi; and an embryonic Farmer Field and Life School project near Pietermaritzburg, South Africa, as reported by Margriet Bredewold, personal communication 10 January 2005).

Altogether it seems however the case that strongly gendered limitations in terms of successful agricultural interventions are women's lack of entitlement to land, housing and other means of production; it has indeed been suggested (even though concrete evidence is scarce) that gender might interact with weak property rights to land and natural resources to diminish incentives for women to adopt higher value crops and environmentally sustainable farming practices (Barnett & Grellier, 2003; Quisumbing et al., 1998).

In addition, even in settings where the introduction of LSTs in agriculture has proven to be successful, who benefits from incurred labour savings is not only household-type specific, but equally related to the gender division of labour. Women in relation to agricultural activities seem to benefit most from technologies that reduce planting and weeding time, while men are said to benefit most from the better use of draught power or tractors (see for example Bishop-Sambrook et al., 2004, in relation to Tanzania). More generally, when LSTs in agriculture are introduced into a context characterized by rigid gender differentiation in combination with unequal access to resources and opportunities for women, this might mean changes in agricultural technology cannot be accessed by women (or only partly), unless more general gender constraints are removed.

It has thus been argued that women would benefit most from domestic LSTs. Even though success rates in the introduction of domestic LSTs have been mixed in the past, many available LSTs - for example hammer mills or other food processing technologies, or community wells and fuel-efficient stoves - do require little further development or testing, and many of those technologies not only benefit individuals or households, but the whole community (Mather et al., 2004b). In addition, in reducing time constraints for household domestic tasks such as food processing, or water and fuel gathering, such domestic LSTs might be a better investment than agriculture-based LSTs in an area hit hard by HIV/AIDS, as they are likely to free time especially for women and girls who are the main care givers for AIDS patients (Mather et al., 2004a). In addition, women are carrying out the majority of tasks associated with social reproduction, including the maintenance of communal institutions and belief systems, and time freed from domestic chores might play an important part in combating an erosion of social capital and socially reproductive labour.[46]

All this leads to a conclusion discussed in more detail in part two of the AWLAE series (Müller, 2005a): What is needed more than anything else is the cultivation of social norms and practices that allow women to exercise control over their lives. In particular poor young women are in need of strategies for building economic and social assets that give them a stronger bargaining position within their families, among their peers, and in sexual relationships (Hallman, 2004).

But a note of caution seems in order here: The persistent need to promote women's access to resources and 'empower' women in every sphere of life raises more general questions about international development endeavours even before the times of AIDS. It is now more than twenty years since awareness of gender analysis and gender issues in development has been raised, having led to a clearer understanding of women's specific vulnerability and having resulted in women having become the target of many development interventions (White, 2002). But looking at past experiences from the vantage point of today, in particular but not only in the light of HIV/AIDS, women often still remain in the same vulnerable position. Development projects have obviously been failing them (White, 2002). Whether increased desperation induced by the progression of the HIV/AIDS pandemic will change that situation is very much open to question. At the end of the day, what is required would be a change in cultural values and myths akin to a revolution.

[46] Social reproduction is not the same as social capital, it has to be noted. Social reproduction is here used to refer to the effort that goes into the reproduction of the social and economic infrastructure (see Barnett & Whiteside, 2002, for further discussion).

It has been documented widely that poor women are those most at risk of HIV infection and least able to mitigate AIDS impact (Farmer, 1996). This would suggest that the alleviation of women's poverty might be an important step on the road towards combating the pandemic. In the wider debate on 'pro-poor' growth it has equally been said that reducing gender inequality in access and control of key resources makes growth more sustainable and 'pro-poor' in the context of sub-Saharan Africa, where gender inequality is a core dimension of poverty (Blackden & Canagarajah, 2003).[47] This leads right back to the introduction to this book: Poverty reinforces HIV/AIDS at all levels and vice versa, and both are exacerbated by gender inequality. Alternatively one can say that gender inequality and HIV/AIDS reinforce each other, and both are exacerbated by poverty. Gender, poverty and more general global inequalities between and within countries and regions stand also in the way of, at present, arguably the best mitigation tool: access to antiretroviral therapy (ART).

[47] Blackden & Canagarajah (2003) cite evidence from Kenya which suggests that if women had the same human capital endowments and used the same amounts of inputs as men, their agricultural output would increase by some twenty-two percent, suggesting women's productivity being well below potential (ibid.:9). Facilitating such gains in productivity by women could thus reduce the level of food insecurity in the region substantially.

5. Antiretroviral treatment as a mitigation tool

Providing access to ART - combined with innovative schemes to address the need for food supplementation within HIV/AIDS treatment programmes and the promotion of other public health services as part of treatment initiatives (Marston & de Cock, 2004; see also Gillespie & Kadiyala, 2005, on the linkages between ART efficiency and nutritional status) - is at present the sole policy intervention that can strengthen resilience and recover capacity. In particular in the countries hardest-hit by HIV/AIDS no other single measure will so quickly arrest the plunge in capacity and allow those countries to 'step back from the edge' (Armstrong, 2003). In due course, treatment is increasingly been regarded as an essential component in the response to the HIV/AIDS pandemic nationally as well as internationally (Shadlen, 2004). It needs to be emphasized here that ART is not a 'magic bullet', it provides mainly a window of opportunity (until, for example, viral resistance might set in). In addition, in a majority of cases ART, even in the form of highly active antiretroviral treatment (HAART) therapies available since the mid-1990s, may delay death for only a few years, while the momentum of population growth in sub-Saharan Africa coupled with the long-wave character of HIV/AIDS will mean rising numbers of death for years to come (UNAIDS, 2005; for an extensive discussion of treatment regimes see Panos Institute, 2000). Having said that, however, to roll out comprehensive ART as widely as possible represents the best window of opportunity currently available. In allowing infected people to live longer and, if accompanied by appropriate diets, to be fully economically productive, treatment gives other measures - including for example agricultural mitigation strategies whether based on LSTs or other means - a chance to work (Barnett & Grellier, 2003; see also Chopra, 2003).[48]

[48] It should be pointed out here that even in the most optimistic scenario anticipated, ART coverage is expected to cover only 70 percent of those in need in sub-Saharan Africa by 2025 - reflecting the fact that upgrading the capacity of existing health systems is a time-consuming and painstaking process (UNAIDS, 2005).

Whereas people at the onset of AIDS-related diseases may only partially withdraw from economic activities, their participation decreases as illnesses become more severe over time, making it impossible not only for the infected person to work but often forcing the carer to equally take time off from productive activities. This withdrawal can be acutely critical not only in the event when disease occurs during peak labour times of the agricultural cycle, but equally when it does so during periods of new technology adoption. ART maintains labour power and with it may allow the timespan needed to make for example LSTs feasible (Bishop-Sambrook, 2003b).

Taken together, ART not only saves lives (at least for the moment) but enables people to remain economically and socially productive, to continue to care for their children, to participate in their communities, and helps to secure the passing of knowledge from generation to generation.

Another effect of access to ART is psychological: With ART, not only the quality of life of an infected person improves considerably, but a future worth living for can be anticipated (again). In settings where ART is becoming more widely available, people understand that AIDS is not an immediate death sentence, but that they can live normally - continue working, interact with family and friends - for an extended period of time if they take proper care of themselves. From the Rakai district in Uganda it has for example been reported that coffin making was a booming business until a few years ago. After the availability of ART brick working started to flourish again, since providing a secure house for their families has become a high priority for infected people (UNAIDS, 2002; see also one of the cases reported in Meinert et al., 2003). Having access to ART thus leads to a different outlook onto the future, modifies the overall "risk environment" (Barnett in Moatti et al., 2003b:253) and may act as a strong incentive for behavioural change (see some of the examples told in Armstrong, 2003; but see Meinert et al., 2003, for the different ways in which ART can impact on individual life worlds).[49] In addition, PLWHA gain social recognition in settings where a government acknowledges their right to treatment and therewith their value to society as a whole (see Galvão, 2002, in relation to Brazil).

It is not only the infected individual, but society at large that benefits from adequate attention to and treatment of HIV/AIDS - it thus seems imperative to suggest that public health policy should give priority to such treatment, also in resource-poor settings, and that in spite of the massive shortage of basic public health infrastructure the "need for antiretroviral therapy in Africa is real and compelling" (Marston & de Cock, 2004:80; see also Collins & Rau, 2000; Mukherjee et al., 2003; Panos Institute, 2000).[50] It has in fact been argued - convincingly in the author's view - that to deny such treatment is not only ethically

[49] In this regard concerns have been raised that improvements in the health status and quality of life of HIV-infected people brought about by ART may indeed increase the opportunities for behaviours that risk HIV transmission and jeopardize prevention efforts. A survey in Côte d'Ivoire shows access to ART not to be associated with HIV-related risky sexual behaviour (Moatti et al., 2003a), while in Tanzania access to care and support (albeit not including ART) has been shown to be associated with increased adoption of preventive behaviour (MacNeil et al., 1999). While undoubtedly more studies will be needed to get a more comprehensive picture of such processes, the data available rather confirm that prevention and access to care, including ART, mutually reinforce each other also in resource-poor settings (Katzenstein et al., 2003; Moatti et al., 2003a; see also the discussion in Blower & Farmer, 2003, on ART as a 'non-conventional prevention tool', and Jones, 2004, on how prevailing representations of Africa skew HIV/AIDS policies towards prevention).

[50] Another concern raised in relation to ART in resource-poor settings is that non-compliance and/or continued unprotected sexual intercourse by people receiving treatment may lead to the transmission of HIV viral strains that have already acquired genetic resistance characteristics against therapies. It is beyond the scope of this publication to discuss those issues in more detail. Evaluations from pilot ART programmes in Côte d'Ivoire, Senegal and Uganda found, however, drug-resistance HIV levels below those in the United States and Europe, thus providing a counter-argument for withholding the diffusion of ART in developing countries (Katzenstein et al., 2003; Moatti et al., 2003a).

contentious and detrimental to public health, but at the same time bad economic policy (see Moatti et al., 2003b).[51]

That prevention, care and treatment generally reinforce each other is a lesson that could have been learned quite early in the global epidemic when looking at the example of Brazil, which shows most clearly the importance of paring prevention with access to treatment (Holden, 2003; Richey & Haakonsson, 2004). Brazil provides a convincing example of the wider benefits incurred through the transformation in the perception of HIV/AIDS from fatal calamity to a manageable disease. Within the framework of the 'Brazilian model', the free distribution of antiretroviral drugs (ARVs) was institutionalized in 1996 and accompanied by voluntary counselling and testing services, the provision of contraceptives, as well as prevention campaigns focusing in particular on young people and sex professionals (Teixeira et al., 2003). This combination of prevention and treatment early on in the epidemic did not only lead to a 80 percent drop in the number of deaths from AIDS related illnesses and vastly fewer new infections than predicted (BBC, 14 July 2003; 18 November 2003; 19

[51] The increasing number of corporations in sub-Saharan Africa that have moved to provide ART for their employees (sometimes including employees' families) at company expense point to the cost-saving potential of such treatment in terms of for example reducing work absenteeism, reducing rehiring and retraining of workers, and retaining a healthier motivated workforce (see Block, 2001; Moatti et al, 2003b; Vermuelen, 2004; also Barnett et al., 2002, for the case of the Debswana mining company in Botswana; Eholie et al., 2003, for the case of the Electricity Company of Côte d'Ivoire; and the website of Journ-AIDS at http://www.journ-aids.org, accessed 18 April 2005, for detailed information on South African companies' responses to HIV/AIDS; but see also Rosen & Simon, 2002, for an observed 'burden-shift' away from the private sector to households and governments). In sharp contrast with those company assessments, major economic arguments made against bridging the North-South gap in access to treatment are still too often based "on a small range of costs defined by particular versions of 'economic' discourse and excluding larger cost associated with lost capacity for social and economic reproduction, non-traded goods and services in the economy and other goods such as 'happiness' and 'well-being'" (Moatti et al. 2003b:249; see also Bujra, 2004, on AIDS and social reproduction).

November 2003; Mukherjee, 2003).[52] It has equally led to a general climate of tolerance and solidarity with those infected (ibid.), thus reducing stigma and exclusion - both of which still a considerable problem in many parts of sub-Saharan Africa (Armstrong, 2003).

It is thus argued here that to hugely expand ART is a moral, social, political and economic imperative, even though the challenges to implementation in most countries in sub-Saharan Africa are unprecedented (Armstrong, 2003; de Waal, 2003).[53] That many sub-Saharan African countries are so ill prepared to meet those challenges is to a large extent a legacy of neo-liberal politics since the 1980s, and Structural Adjustment Programmes (SAPs) that have left many African countries with scaled down social service delivery systems and more generally eroded the foundations for improving state-capacity (Bujra, 2004; Lurie et al., 2004; Richey & Haakonsson, 2004).

But over the last years evidence has emerged in relation to successful ART programmes in developing countries or resource-poor settings (Katzenstein et al., 2003).[54] In addition to the case of Brazil (Galvão,

[52] New HIV infections in Brazil fell from 24,816 in 1998 to just 7361 in the first nine months of 2001 (Mukherjee, 2003). The total number of PLWHA in Brazil in 2003 was estimated at 610,000. In 1992, the World Bank had predicted that without intervention 1.2 million Brazilians would be HIV positive by 2000 (BBC, 14 July 2003; Teixeira et al., 2003). Interestingly, it was twenty years ago that Brazil and South Africa both registered their first AIDS cases, in Sao Paulo and Johannesburg respectively. In South Africa the government neglected the spread of HIV for many years with the result that in 2003 more than 4.7 million South Africans were infected.

[53] The most 'successful' scenario for the future - in terms of curbing the HIV/AIDS pandemic - narrated by UNAIDS (2005) equally has a strong focus on the safe delivery of ART which will lead gradually to the expansion of health care systems and the broadening of civil society skills and engagement. This focus on ART is to be combined with sustained investment in infrastructure as well as a transformation in the structural and development issues that fuel the pandemic in Africa, including the global regimes of aid and trade, poverty, and gender relations (UNAIDS, 2005).

[54] Gray et al. (2003) argue in this respect that ART alone is insufficient to control the spread of HIV in settings where the epidemic is mature, and the number of people in need of ART will increase over time. ART in combination with a low efficacy vaccine, however, could control the epidemic if behavioural disinhibition is prevented at the same time. They conclude that while improved access to ART is needed for eligible HIV-infected people in developing countries to improve survival and quality of life, there is at the same time a need to consider the societal benefits of therapy in terms of overall control of the HIV epidemic.

2002; Teixeira et al., 2003), the feasibility of ART and its potential to successfully treat large numbers of HIV-infected patients has been demonstrated for example in under-privileged areas of Malawi (Durier, 2003), in Côte d'Ivoire (Djomand et al., 2003), in Senegal (Desclaux et al., 2002; Laurent et al., 2002) and in Haiti (expanding on experiences with directly-observed therapy (DOT) in relation to tuberculosis treatment, see Farmer et al., 2001; see also UNAIDS, 1997, for a general discussion of a dual strategy to fight HIV/AIDS and tuberculosis).[55]

As one of the most difficult challenges in ART pilot projects in the developing world the need for a clear political and financial commitment not only from the national government and local medical community, but equally from donor organisations (and their governments) and the pharmaceutical industry has been identified (Djomand et al., 2003). More generally it has been argued that the global context of aid and trade needs to be altered to eventually arrive at feasible treatment regimes in sub-Saharan Africa,[56] particularly so in the light of the protection offered to the pharmaceutical industry under the intellectual property regime enacted with the Trade-Related Aspects of Intellectual Property Rights (TRIPS) agreement in 1994 (for a more detailed discussion of TRIPS and its potential consequences for AIDS-policy see Orsi et al., 2003).

It has been estimated that from the more than 39 million people infected with HIV to date, 5.8 million are in need of ART, much more than the three by five campaign envisages to provide (UNAIDS/WHO, 2004; WHO, 2003).[57] Looking at Africa as a region, in 2003 just two

[55] Small pilot studies on ART for HIV-2 infected people, a strain less common and less virulent, suggest that while in contrast to HIV-1 only a limited number of ART options show a positive response, with a well-chosen treatment regime sustained viral suppression can also be achieved for HIV-2 patients (see Adjé-Touré et al., 2003; van der Ende et al., 2003).

[56] While the author totally agrees with that point, to discuss it in more detail is beyond the scope of this publication; but see the discussion in Love (2004), Richey & Haakonsson (2004) and Shadlen (2004).

[57] Looking at the example of Uganda, a country receiving substantial international funds for its AIDS programmes with a large share of that money earmarked for treatment, it has been estimated that by 2007 as a best-case scenario 100,000 Ugandans might be on treatment, but 150,000 would be in need of it (Feuer, 2004).

percent of the people estimated in need of ART had access to such treatment, a number that had risen to eight percent by December 2004 - compared to 65 percent in the Americas, the latter largely reflecting the success of Brazil (WHO, 2003; http://www.who.int/3by5, accessed 21 March 2005). This points to one of the key challenges for national treatment campaigns, access to affordable medication. It has been argued that the main impetus behind Brazil's large-scale public treatment access policy was the drive to set up a strategy for reducing prices for ARVs (Orsi et al., 2003). The success of the 'Brazilian model' was strongly related to Brazil putting pressure on pharmaceutical companies that if they would not reduce the price of patented anti-retroviral drugs (ARVs), Brazil would allow cheap copies of those drugs to be imported or produce generic drugs on its own (BBC, 23 August 2001; 06 September 2003). Brazil was in a position to apply this pressure because it has the scientific and economic resources to carry out this 'threat' and use the mechanism of 'compulsory licensing';[58] and it already produced some of the non patent protected drugs in the ARV cocktail locally (Bellos, 2001; Teixeira, et al., 2003). The Brazilian government subsequently managed to negotiate the desired discounts from all pharmaceutical companies whose drugs are used in the country's ART programme (ibid.; BBC, 18 November 2003; see also the discussion in Orsi et al., 2003; Shadlen, 2004).[59]

Apart from the key challenge for national treatment campaigns to secure a stable and reliable flow of drugs at affordably prices into the long term future (see Shadlen, 2004, for an extensive discussion of those

[58] Compulsory licensing is a stipulation incorporated into TRIPS in the Doha Declaration approved by the World Trade Organisation (WTO) in November 2001. It allows specifically authorised copying of patented drugs in the event of a health emergency, albeit with a number of restrictions imposed on the issuing country (see Orsi et al., 2003, for a more extensive discussion). To the knowledge of the author, thus far no compulsory licence measures have been taken by the Brazilian government (see Orsi et al., 2003, for a discussion of the obstacles faced by Brazil in issuing such licences).

[59] A similar victory was scored by the South African Treatment Action Campaign (TAC) in securing imports of certain generic drugs or the rights to in-country production (Armstrong, 2003). It was mainly fear of possible damage done to their global reputation that made the pharmaceutical companies give in eventually. For a more general discussion of treatment regimes, including first- and second-line treatment, HAART, and generic fixed-dose combinations of ARVs, see Christian Aid (2004); Panos Institute (2000).

two issues),[60] ART thus raises more general questions about distribution, about the policy decisions that have to be made in terms of who gets access to free treatment via the public health services.[61] Provision of ART shows the need for a capable state with the goal of health equity, including equity of access in terms of gender, rural-urban residency and poverty, and the means to enforce such goals, either by government degree or, ideally, by involving communities in defining priorities for treatment access (see Richey & Haakonsson, 2004; Moatti et al., 2003b, on successful community involvement in Uganda and South Africa; but also Gruber & Caffrey, 2005, on how donor-funded HIV/AIDS activities can lead to community conflict). Looking at Brazil again as the first developing country to have implemented a large-scale ART programme, its experience was based on what is considered 'best practice' - a concerted government response coupled with the effective participation of civil society (Teixeira et al., 2003).

Such a response also needs long-term funding commitments, something international donors, who will have to contribute substantially to make treatment a reality in most of sub-Saharan Africa, are usually reluctant to give, and a health system geared towards the treatment of chronic

[60] A new potential obstacle in securing access to ART in developing countries emerges as this book goes in print: From 2005 India has to comply with the new international law being set up under TRIPS. In March 2005 India was thus in the process of issuing a new patent law that is bound to change the availability of cheap generic versions of patented ARVs (under the old law, Indian drug makers were allowed to copy patented drugs as long as they used a different manufacturing process). An estimated 50 percent of people receiving ART in the developing world are said to depend on generic drugs from India. It is feared that the new Indian law will decrease the production of generic ARVs and push up prices for ART. How far WTO regulations - allowing for some leeway in cases of serious epidemics such as AIDS - will still allow Indian firms to export generic drugs to developing countries without indigenous manufacturing facilities, as well as how much the enforcement of patent rights may undermine the ability of governments like Brazil's to negotiate cheaper prices with multinational pharmaceutical companies remains to be seen (see BBC, 18 March 2003; BBC, 22 March 2003; Orsi et al., 2003).

[61] One such issue which has aroused considerable debate is the practice of prioritising the use of ART for prevention of mother-to-child transmission without giving continuing treatment to mothers who are sick, thus protecting the baby while its untreated mother is left to die. While short-course regimens for prevention of mother-to-child transmission have been shown to be cost-effective (Freedberg & Yazdanpanah, 2003), treatment of HIV positive mothers should be as imperative to any comprehensive health strategy (see Mukherjee et al., 2003). See also Schaffer & Lamb (1974) on a general discussion of 'the problem of access', discussed in terms of the relations between the administrative allocation of goods and services and the people for whom they are intended.

diseases, which most developing countries' systems are not. But those challenges - often used as a pretext for focusing public health interventions exclusively on prevention (Laurent et al., 2002) - are no justification for a lack of engagement by the international community nor by national or local activists, as the examples of successes show and moral imperatives demand. They do call for a scaling up of the response, and a shift from the current dominant emphasis on the provision of drugs towards building adequate systems of delivery combined with mechanisms to secure reliable access to affordable supplies (Richey & Haakonsson, 2004; Sheldon, 2004).[62]

Taken together, bringing ART to all who need it will require an adequately funded functioning health system at national, regional, district and village level - small-scale replications of successful NGO projects, whether local or foreign, often depending on donor funding and agendas, are insufficient to meet national health needs (Bujra, 2004; Sachs, 2005). To lay the foundations for such a health system is altogether a long term and expensive task, but a task that would address the character of HIV/AIDS as a metaphor for development gone wrong, as such health systems would more generally contribute to the public health of thus far marginalized populations (see for example the discussion in Jones, 2004). One of the major obstacles in health care infrastructure is the lack of trained personnel with appropriate experience (see for example Armstrong, 2003), which, together with all the other constraints facing adequate public health provision can only be overcome with systematic policy and planning, for which local and global political leadership and strong government commitment is a necessary (if not sufficient) condition (Sachs, 2005).[63] More generally, looking at public health policies and programmes, these need

[62] Shadlen (2004) argues in this context that unaffordable drug prices can serve as a disincentive to invest in healthcare infrastructure that is essential for treatment, while low prices can create incentives to build such an infrastructure (see also Berwick, 2002).

[63] The absurdity in the way international development assistance works comes to the fore here once again: While on one hand Uganda receives a flood of money for its ART programme it is lacking trained providers with appropriate experiences. At the same time, the World Bank has imposed a hiring freeze on the Ministry of Health - even though the Bank itself is loaning money for ART programmes (Feuer, 2004). More generally, many African countries too poor to invest in AIDS treatment and prevention have been congratulated for successes in macro-economic stabilisation while life expectancies have turned deeply downwards (Sachs, 2005).

some rigour to succeed and need to be accompanied by compliance procedures. The latter is difficult to advocate in times in which participation and civil society are en vogue and state imposed programmes find little favour with the donor community (de Waal, 2003; see also the discussion in Putzel, 2003).

It should be noted that ART is not advocated here as a replacement for strategies to prevent the spread of the pandemic and mitigate its non-health impact. In the light of the absence of an effective vaccine, without which long term control of the epidemic will be impossible even in settings where prevention and treatment measures have been implemented successfully like in Brazil, and considering the challenge of providing ART within existing infrastructures in poor countries, wider mitigation must remain a top priority in any pro-poor policy for the rural sector and beyond (see Allison & Seeley, 2004; Teixeira et al., 2003; and the website of the International AIDS Vaccine Initiative at http://www.iavi.org, accessed 18 April 2005, for up-to-date information on all issues around vaccine development).[64]

[64] For a different line of argument in the discussion on ART see Page (2001) who argues that an integrated effort to address the wider needs of rural HIV infected women is a more cost-effective and feasible strategy than making ART more widely available.

6. Conclusion

The preceding discussion suggests a number of lessons to be learned if HIV/AIDS mitigation is to be (more) successful in the future.

Firstly, continued support for national poverty reduction is crucial for sustainable mitigation, combined with more general efforts to address the developmental impact of the epidemic. Looking at rural livelihoods, the causes and manifestations of impoverishment as a factor in HIV transmission need to be better understood for different agricultural systems and livelihoods. Many of the shocks that have befallen rural livelihoods have indeed been a direct consequence of development paradigms pursued by international donor agencies - the most prominent being SAPs (for a detailed discussion of the various links between SAPs and HIV/AIDS see Collins & Rau, 2000; Lurie et al., 2004; Schoepf, 2004). Others reflect structural factors that have made societies and specific groups within society vulnerable to conditions conducive to HIV transmission, including the global political economy and market forces.[65]

Ultimately, a new paradigm for development is asked for, a paradigm that combines social protection and development, is based on people's own perceptions and priorities, and explicitly addresses the key structural factors driving the epidemic, two of the most important of which are poverty and gender inequalities (Kim et al., 2002). Only a symbiosis between longer-standing social agendas on for example education, food security, local democracy on the one hand and HIV/AIDS mitigation on the other will allow both sets of targets to be

[65] Malawi serves as a good example here: In Malawi, rural farming households have historically functioned as long-distance male labour reserves - at first for South African mines, later for Malawi's plantations - bringing with it a strict gender division of labour and dual character to household labour efforts, with great reliance on cash income by men from distant places (see Bryceson et al., 2004; Munthali, 2002). During the course of the last years the male migrant labour system has been disintegrating, with adverse repercussions for rural cash flows. During a famine that hit Malawi in 2001-2002 the formerly cushioning effect of migrant labour remittances was largely absent, leading to widely reported cases of women and girls exchanging sex for basic foodstuffs (Bryceson et al., 2004).

met (de Waal, 2003).[66] For both, national leadership, political courage and international support are needed. More generally, the devastating effect AIDS has on African societies highlights the need for public goods, not least a health system capable of administering complex public health programmes, that only governments - whether acting unilaterally or multilaterally - can provide (Boone & Batsell, 2001; Fukuyama, 2004). Ultimately, the still dominant biomedical model that incorporates "capitalist economic assumptions about health resulting from individually chosen lifestyles" (Schoepf, 2004:18) needs to be replaced by a concept of public health where health is regarded as a "public rather than an individual responsibility" (ibid.).

Secondly, mitigation interventions should not be tailored to target HIV/AIDS afflicted and affected households or PLWHA in particular. Apart from the ethical implications involved in such targeting in an environment where stigma against PLWHA often prevails, not all afflicted households or individuals are equally affected, while the poor who are not affected (yet) might be equally in need of social assistance. Targeting should thus be done according to different indicators (see for example Aliber et al., 2004; O'Donnell, 2004). Research to date shows that poor strata of rural households headed by widows, grandparents or orphans are the most vulnerable, and it has thus been argued that AIDS impact mitigation should centre on 'pro-poor' and gender-sensitive growth while assistance in the form of resource transfers should centre on households with few alternative sources of support (Lundberg & Over, 2000; Mather et al., 2004b; White, 2002; see also Nyamukapa & Gregson, 2005, on programme assistance for different groups of orphans, and Sauerborn et al., 1996, on a more general discussion of targeting of special health services towards certain categories of households).

The need for a more comprehensive than strictly HIV/AIDS centred response also emerges from people's own perceptions. A survey by Afrobarometer conducted across fifteen countries, including the high

[66] As one way to achieve such a symbiosis it has been suggested that interventions must be considered across the full spectrum of the sustainable livelihoods framework - see Harvey (2003) who provides a comprehensive discussion outlining possible responses in relation to all aspects of livelihood.

HIV prevalence countries in southern and eastern Africa, found that even in the latter support for prioritising anti-AIDS spending over other social spending was rather a minority position. Among people living in poverty HIV/AIDS connected spending was even less considered a priority, as they face too many other problems (Afrobarometer, April 2004, http://www.afrobarometer.org, accessed 24 February 2005).[67] More generally it has indeed been argued that one should not underestimate the general disillusionment of in particular rural populations for whom HIV/AIDS is just an additional ailment, often less immediate than the daily survival (Collins & Rau, 2000; see also Aliber et al., 2004, on HIV/AIDS being 'just another way of dying'; and Sauerborn et al., 1996, on household priorities at times of ill health).[68]

Thirdly, the main conclusion drawn from what has been said so far here is that successful interventions and mitigation strategies will only be sustainable if they are aimed not only at households and individuals, but ultimately address the wider community and society, and foster what has been called 'social cohesion'. Social cohesion can be defined as 'a sense of solidarity and common purpose' (Maxwell, 2003). Looking at the various epidemics in Africa, the case can be made that high incidence of HIV is associated with poor social cohesion (Decosas, 2002; see also the general discussion on social epidemiology in Krieger, 2001).

[67] Those findings are in line with the experiences of a Master's student in Management of Agro-ecological Knowledge and Social Change (MAKS) at Wageningen University, whose thesis is attached to a farmer field and life school project in Msinga district in KwaZulu Natal in South Africa. She found people simply had more urgent day-to-day problems to be too much concerned about HIV/AIDS in a community where awareness is high and some PLWHA are having access to ART through the public health system (personal communication with Margriet Bredewold, 10 January 2005).

[68] One should take note here that less poverty alone is not necessarily bound to make a difference in terms of the spread of the pandemic, if not coupled with awareness of the dynamics of AIDS-related vulnerability. Much of the impact of the pandemic is invisible for quite a long time, so people need to understand those linkages and dynamics (and it is here that interventions such as FLSs can have an important function). On the other hand, it has for example been reported from Malawi that the biggest constraint farming households, be they AIDS afflicted or affected or not, face, is the high cost of fertilizer and the removal of fertilizer subsidies in the course of SAP measures is seen as devastating - and may indirectly be one of the reasons behind increasing rates of transactional sexual encounters (see Bryceson et al., 2004). In this context the reintroduction of a redistributive measure (fertilizer subsidies) could potentially alleviate the situation for many farmers while making farm households less susceptible and vulnerable to HIV/AIDS.

In contrast, societies characterized by strong social cohesion, even if they are poor, have thus far experienced comparatively lower levels of HIV prevalence (Barnett, Whiteside & Decosas, 2000; see also Müller, 2005b).[69] Countries can be "classified as being more or less socially cohesive on the basis of the distribution of income, the level of ethnic or social tension, [or] the presence of strong conformist (...) religions, ideologies [or] political regimes" (Decosas, 2002:9). Islam as a highly controlling framework has for example been associated with the lower HIV prevalence rate in most predominately Muslim countries (see Gray, 2004, for a discussion of available studies on the relationship between HIV and Islam, suggesting that Islamic religious affiliation is indeed negatively associated with HIV seropositivity).[70] A similar argument has been made in connection with some protestant churches. Research in South Africa and Zimbabwe has revealed that people belonging to 'spirit-type' churches (for example the Pentecostal church), characterized by restrictive social norms and a high degree of internal observation, are less susceptible to HIV infection (Garner, 2000; Gregson et al., 1999).[71]

People-centred political ideologies - in particular when accompanied by a social revolution - and the governance structures often accompanying those can have a similar effect in advancing social solidarity, while at the same time fostering behavioural norms negatively correlated with HIV transmission. This may for example

[69] One needs to point out here that while social cohesion may be the result of good governance and a strong civil society, it can equally be the product of control or repression under a hegemonic ideology (see Barnett, Whiteside & Decosas, 2000). Strongly repressive societies might indeed show the same 'epidemiological advantages' as strongly cohesive societies (see Decosas, 2002); once this repression ends, there might then occur a rapid shift towards the opposite risk pattern.

[70] AWLAE scholar Aifa Ndoye, whose research topic is 'Analysis of micro-economic and macro-economic performance of market gardening production in Senegal within a context of low HIV/AIDS prevalence' made a similar point in her presentation at a HIV/AIDS policy workshop held at Wageningen University on 25 October 2004: In addition to enlightened government policies, she regards the moral framework offered by Islam as decisive in Senegal's success in keeping HIV prevalence low.

[71] A slightly weaker connection between religious affiliation (of any kind) and HIV/AIDS has been documented from Ghana. A study found that such affiliation, through fostering social networks, improves the diffusion of knowledge on HIV/AIDS particularly among women; it does not, however, show any effect in terms of behavioural change (Takyi, 2003).

explain the rapid fall in HIV prevalence in post-revolutionary Uganda, as well as the low prevalence rate in post-revolutionary Eritrea (see Decosas, 2002; Müller, 2004b; 2005a; 2005b). In the absence of such social solidarity, to facilitate behavioural change might have to rely on compliance procedures, on what could be called "inclusive authoritarianism" (UNAIDS, 2005:70) - such compliance procedures have in fact also been reported from (relatively) socially cohesive Uganda and Cuba (see Allen & Heald, 2004; Putzel, 2004, and the discussion in Müller, 2005b). Following this line of thought it has been argued that HIV/AIDS in the context of sub-Saharan Africa needs to be redefined as a 'public health and infectious disease emergency' (de Cock et al., 2002), with all the necessary policies and practices that this might entail, including for example partner notification and an increased focus on treatment (ibid.).[72]

Those findings have implications for HIV/AIDS mitigation strategies, no matter whether they take place in urban settings or rural environments, on a societal scale or in relation to certain sub-groups or communities. They suggest the strengthening of community-based organisations that are dedicated to social equity and mutual caring and support as one of the main pillars of HIV competence and AIDS mitigation, not prevention messages per se that might not have much to do with the lived realities of many highly susceptible populations (Decosas, 2002; see also Allen & Heald, 2004 on why policies succeeded in Uganda but failed in Botswana; and Donahue, 1998, on supporting the creation of community safety nets). Such organisations and networks are bound to increase social cohesion at the communal level and possibly beyond and therewith reduce people's susceptibility to HIV infection. A study conducted in rural eastern Zimbabwe for example argues that cohesive social networks may provide "contexts for the development of a sense of comradeship and solidarity which

[72] To date, human-rights-based approaches to HIV/AIDS prevention, adopted from early AIDS policies in the United States and western Europe and based on an understanding of human rights biased towards civil and political, rather than social and economic ones (see Jones, 2004), have often rather undermined public health approaches and reduced the importance of social justice. See also Manning (2002) where it is argued that while higher levels of social cohesion might help to contain the epidemic, democratisation does not necessarily increase such cohesion but might turn out to be detrimental to it.

may boost members' confidence, social skills, and sense of perceived self-efficacy", and ultimately "supportive contexts within which peers can make collectively negotiated decisions to change their behaviour" (Gregson et al., 2004:2121). It corresponds with findings from Uganda - in contrast to a number of southern African countries - which show that one major determinant of the behavioural profile of a population is the personalisation of risk, and in the case of Uganda a unique shift has occurred from impersonal (media) to personal channels for communicating about AIDS between 1985 and 1995 (Low-Beer & Stoneburner, 2003; see also the study by Smith & Watkins, 2005, on local social networks as an important mechanism for identifying sources of risk and developing strategies to prevent HIV/AIDS in Malawi). More generally, HIV/AIDS can have a positive impact on social cohesion if it makes people and communities join forces together to face the collective challenges brought about by the pandemic (Loewenson & Whiteside, 2001; UNAIDS, 2005).

Creating greater community cohesiveness or networks of social solidarity might thus be one of the most important approaches to shifting the risk profile of a population and ultimately mitigating the impact of HIV/AIDS, as well as for making treatment campaigns more successful (Collins & Rau, 2000; Decosas, 2002). In socially-cohesive settings, individualism and the values of the market are restrained by 'social morality' (Collins & Rau, 2000).[73] A focus on social cohesion and communal networks is of particular relevance to the African context, about which it has been said not only that "Africa's strength lies in social networks which are invisible to many outsiders", but also that while development "in the West" is "about increasing choice for individuals, in Africa it is more about increasing human dignity *within a community*" (Commission for Africa, 2005:26; *my emphasis*).

This discussion brings us back to the first point raised in these concluding remarks: Dealing with HIV/AIDS in sub-Saharan Africa will

[73] See also the discussion in Beeker et al. (1998) on community empowerment as an intervention framework in the context of the United States, where it is argued that the community empowerment paradigm not only widens one's lens to include the social and structural context in which HIV transmission occurs, but equally pays attention to selecting intervention strategies that are compatible with a community's stage of readiness.

more than anything else require a vigorous, developmentalist response on part of the African state, as such a state is necessary to lay the foundations for the creation of a civil society that fosters, rather then inhibits, social solidarity (Boone & Batsell, 2001; Putzel, 2004).[74] Such processes require a significant amount of social and political capital (on top of financial resources, see Low-Beer & Stoneburner, 2003), an inclusive strategy pursued by the political leadership of the day based on broad social mobilisation, and a new kind of interaction between state and civil society (Moran, 2004; Schoepf, 2003; see also Teixeira et al., 2003, on the case of Brazil; and Price-Smith & Daly, 2004, on how the absence of such a strategy has undermined state capacity and resulted in manifold political conflicts in Zimbabwe).

Ultimately, the success of mitigating the impact of the HIV/AIDS pandemic will, however, also rest on the international community and the workings of the global political economy, not least in achieving a more just distribution of ART, but also in arriving at new relations between African governments, donor countries and other development partners, a relationship in which African governments themselves determine the way they wish to go and the policies they wish to pursue, coupled with changes in global trade regimes (see for example the discussion in Fredland, 1998; and Commission for Africa, 2005, in particular on aid, debt, and donor-relations).

All these issues are high on the international agenda at the time of writing, pushed by the British government as current chair of the G8 group of industrialised nations and laid out in comprehensive detail in the Report of the Commission for Africa published in March 2005. The report is addressed to the international community in the light of the G8 summit in July 2005, the UN summit reviewing progress made on the MDGs in New York in September 2005, and the World Trade Organisation (WTO) meeting in Hong Kong in December 2005. Sub-Saharan Africa will be the benchmark for measuring success and failure of the international development agenda, and a decisive determinant of success will depend on the national and global policies of action on

[74] Looking at the example of Uganda again, it has often been overlooked that "the central state was pivotal, not only in creating the space for the associational sector to act, but in initially mobilising the sector around HIV/AIDS" (Putzel, 2004:27).

HIV/AIDS. The Commission for Africa Report - while merging recommendations for action on HIV/AIDS with those for action on education, basic health, and water and sanitation - does acknowledge as much in stating that "there is a powerful case for placing and resourcing the response to HIV and AIDS in a special category over and above the other challenges of development" (Commission for Africa, 2005:86). Which of the three scenarios outlined by UNAIDS (2005) for the future of Africa will the world live to see in 2025? If Africa is to 'overcome' and not to remain 'trapped' in a downward spiral of poverty, economic decline, social unrest and political instability, 'though choices' have to be taken today to mitigate the impact of the HIV/AIDS pandemic, halt its spread, and in due course give human development a chance.

Part 2 – Annotated bibliography

1. HIV/AIDS, poverty, development, social cohesion and public health

Allen, T. and S. **Heald** (2004) 'HIV/AIDS Policy in Africa: What has worked in Uganda and what has failed in Botswana?', *Journal of International Development* **16**, pp. 1141-1154.

This paper compares the HIV/AIDS policies pursued in Uganda and Botswana in order to shed light on the kinds of policies that are necessary to contain the epidemic in sub-Saharan Africa. It is suggested that a crucial factor explaining the failure of early programmes in Botswana and the relative success of such programmes in Uganda relates to condom promotion. Such promotion - initially absent in Uganda - has provoked antipathy from church groups, local healers, parents and traditional chiefs in Botswana, undermining a wider social acceptance of behavioural change messages. Other important factors contributing to Uganda's success are identified as leadership at local and national level, community mobilization, as well as economic incentives to contain the spread of the epidemic. In addition, in parts of Uganda sexual behavioural change has been enforced by compliance mechanisms at community level. The paper ends with calling in general for more draconian public health measures than those currently propagated in a situation like that in some sub-Saharan African countries where the epidemic has become endemic.

Barnett, T. and A. **Whiteside** (2002) 'Poverty and HIV/AIDS: Impact, Coping and Mitigation Policy', in G. A. Cornia (ed.) *AIDS, Public Policy and Child Well-Being*, Chapter 11. Florence: UNICEF. http://www.unicef-icdc.org/research/ESP/aids/chapter11.pdf, accessed 18 April 2005.

This book chapter discusses the relation between HIV/AIDS and poverty as well as the relation between poverty and HIV/AIDS, the latter issue being characterized by a lack of conclusive or persuasive research. Important findings include: HIV/AIDS has to be viewed as a development crisis, a crisis that deepens poverty and increases inequality at every level, from the household to the global, a crisis that has for example reversed progress towards the MDGs. The language of 'coping' has to be questioned in relation to HIV/AIDS impact, as many households and communities might indeed not be coping. While there exists an overall lack of documentation of mitigation strategies (apart from a few studies at the communal or household level), it needs to be acknowledged that the epidemic has social roots and thus needs a social - in addition to a medical and technical - response. As a step towards improving the documentation of interventions the chapter ends with a listing of mainly NGO-driven interventions in sub-Saharan Africa and outlines their activities in some detail.

Barnett, T., A. **Whiteside** and J. **Decosas** (2000) 'The Jaipur Paradigm - A Conceptual Framework for Understanding Social Susceptibility and Vulnerability to HIV', *Journal of the South African Medical Association* **90**, pp. 1098-1101.

The so-called Jaipur Paradigm starts from the fact that the profiles of local HIV epidemics vary remarkably. Those differences in epidemic profiles between different societies or communities are thought to depend on underlying social, economic and cultural factors. The paradigm proposes two variables to determine susceptibility and vulnerability of a society to HIV, and thus the likely epidemic profile. These are (1) the degree of social cohesion and (2) the overall level of wealth of a society. In combining the two variables, the categorisation of societies and communities into four broad 'types', each with a distinct HIV prevalence pattern, is facilitated - these patterns are (1) high social cohesion and high wealth, (2) low social cohesion and high wealth, (3) low social cohesion and low wealth and (4) high social cohesion and low wealth. Country examples for each pattern are provided. The paradigm means to draw attention to the fact that social interventions to curb the epidemic need to address 'social development issues' like equality, human rights and the construction of 'civil society'. The applicability and usefulness of the paradigm and its underlying concepts need to be tested in more detailed case studies from which it can then be refined.

Beegle, K. (2003) *Labour Effects of Adult Mortality in Tanzanian Households*. World Bank Policy Research Paper **3062**. Washington DC: World Bank.

This paper, based on panel data from Kagera region in Tanzania, examines how prime-age adult mortality affects the time allocation of surviving household members and the portfolio of household farming activities. Analysis of farm and chore hours across different demographic groups generally found only small and insignificant changes in labour supply of individuals in households experiencing a prime-age adult death. Some farming activities were temporarily scaled back and wage employment fell after a male death. But overall, households did not shift cultivation towards subsistence farming nor did they appear to have reduced their income diversification more than six months after such a death had occurred.

Bell, C., S. **Devarajan** and H. **Gersbach** (2004) 'Thinking About the Long-run Economic Costs of AIDS', in M. Haacker (ed.) *The Macroeconomics of HIV/AIDS*, Washington DC: International Monetary Fund (IMF).

This chapter argues that AIDS has the potential to transform societies by undermining the transfer of human capital from one generation to the next, arguably the core mechanism by which societies flourish. In being a fatal disease of young adults, AIDS makes it difficult for these adults to provide for the education of their children. The result is potentially a generation of under-educated and unproductive Youth who in adulthood will find it difficult to provide for the education of their children, and so forth. In this way, when hit by an HIV/AIDS epidemic, an otherwise growing economy could spiral downwards into a low-level subsistence economy in a few generations. This potential collapse will not be felt immediately. Estimates of economic impact of AIDS that look only at the short to medium term effects of a reduction in labour supply are thus regarded as dangerously misleading. The paper argues that it is, however, possible to avert a downward spiral, but only with aggressive policies aimed at shoring up the faltering mechanisms of human capital transmission between generations. Such policies need to prevent the further spread of HIV/AIDS, prolong the lives of those already infected, and support the education of its victims' children. Such policies - it is argued - might seem expensive in the short term, but when viewed against a possible economic collapse in the longer term, in all likelihood combined with a collapse of society itself, they seem like a bargain.

Collins, J. and B. **Rau** (2000) *AIDS in the Context of Development*. UNRISD Programme on Social Policy and Development, Paper No. **4**. Geneva: United Nations Research Institute for Social Development (UNRISD).

This paper sets out to provide the background for new comparative research on HIV/AIDS as a problem of development. Moving away from an epidemiological or behavioural focus on the pandemic, it begins by discussing AIDS in the context of worsening poverty. Two strategies adopted by poor people in an attempt to secure a livelihood that are at the same time particularly conducive to the spread of HIV/AIDS are discussed in some detail: migration and sex-work. The paper then discusses the series of other shocks that during the past decades have exacerbated often already precarious living conditions for large numbers of people in particular in the developing world, making them more susceptible to disease in general and HIV infection in particular. Those include natural disasters, debt crises, and structural adjustment programmes, the latter two often a direct outcome of development paradigms pursued by international donor agencies. Looking at responses to the pandemic, the critical role of NGOs and community groups is highlighted in providing examples of such responses, while responses formulated by public health departments and donor agencies are critically examined. A central conclusion of the study is the importance of networks of social solidarity and broad-based political action if the pandemic is to be brought under control. The paper ends with suggestions for further social science research on HIV/AIDS and development, so that HIV/AIDS can be integrated into international debates on major development issues - something too often missing.

Decosas, J. (2002) 'The Social Ecology of AIDS in Africa'. Geneva: United Nations Research Institute for Social Development (UNRISD).

This draft paper - expanding on the propositions of the 'Jaipur Paradigm' (see Barnett, Whiteside & Decosas, 2000) as well as on the work of Wilkinson (1996) - is based on an ecological analysis of the HIV/AIDS epidemic in Africa. Social cohesion in its various forms is defined as a crucial determinant of a community's (and with it an individual's) susceptibility and vulnerability to the epidemic. It is thus argued that HIV/AIDS requires community targeted interventions instead of the prevailing focus on behavioural change of individuals, as with such interventions the risk profile of a population is bound to change: they increase social cohesion and thereby reduce a population's susceptibility. Other issues raised include how to 'measure' such cohesion and it is suggested that an important focus should be on communities and sub-groups rather than or in addition to on society as a whole.

Garner, R. (2000) 'Safe sects? dynamic religion and AIDS in Southern Africa', *The Journal of Modern African Studies* **38**, pp. 41-69.

Based on research in the township of Edendale in KwaZulu in South Africa, an area with high HIV prevalence, the article presents evidence on the level of extra- and premarital sex among members of different church types. It is argued that only among members of one of the 'dynamic' churches, the Pentecostal church - which demands and receives a high level of commitment from its members and exercises a high degree of ideological power through indoctrination, religious experience, exclusion, and socialisation - extra- and premarital sexual activities were considerably lower than among non-church goers or members of other Christian denominations. These findings seem to indicate that value-free education which only communicates the dangers of infection is largely ineffectual when not accompanied by a value-laden discourse that makes sexual relations outside marriage opprobrious, and a closed social environment which exerts a credible threat of disciplinary action in the event of 'sin' (see also Gregson et. al, 1999).

Gillespie, S. and S. **Kadiyala** (2005) *HIV/AIDS and Food and Nutrition Security. From Evidence to Action*. Food Policy Review **7**. Washington DC: International Food Policy Research Institute (IFPRI).

This report is a review of existing research into the linkages between HIV/AIDS, food security and nutrition security. The potential impact of food- and nutrition insecurity on the spread of HIV is discussed as well as the impact of HIV/AIDS on food and nutrition security, a discussion that basically repeats points argued before by the same and other authors working at the International Food Policy Research Institute (see for example Gillespie et al., 2001). In line with those previous publications, responses are outlined and the application of an 'HIV/AIDS lens' is advocated (see Müller, 2004a for further details and references). What makes the publication still useful is the two part annex presenting an 'Evidence Base' on HIV/AIDS and food security and HIV/AIDS and nutrition respectively, where available studies are listed and their key findings and recommendations presented.

Gregson, S., N. **Terceira**, P. **Mushati**, C. **Nyamukapa** and C. **Campbell** (2004) 'Community group participation: Can it help young women to avoid HIV? An exploratory study of social capital and school education in rural Zimbabwe', *Social Science and Medicine* **58**, pp. 2119-2132.

This paper starts from the assumption that participatory programmes which address underlying structural and community level factors are essential to reduce the risk of HIV infection in particular for women in rural and urban southern Africa. It then uses cross-sectional data from a large-scale population-based survey in rural eastern Zimbabwe to describe the relationship between membership in different types of community groups and young women's chances of avoiding HIV. Findings include that participation in local community groups is indeed often positively associated with successful avoidance of HIV infection which in turn is positively associated with safe behaviour. This two-way relationship does, however, depend on a number of factors such as the functioning of the group, its purpose, as well as the educational level of the group's participants - the latter seemingly an important factor in determining the social capital value of community groups in relation to HIV prevention. While the paper acknowledges that longitudinal studies are needed to explore those relationships in more details, it is equally suggested that the promotion of and organisational development among community groups could be an effective HIV control strategy.

Gregson, S., T. **Zhuwau**, R. **Anderson** and S. **Chandiwana** (1999) 'Apostles and Zionists: The influence of religion on demographic change in rural Zimbabwe', *Population Studies* **53**, pp. 179-193.

The article describes a study in two rural areas of Zimbabwe, the Honde and Rusitu valleys in the eastern province of Manicaland respectively, which found substantial differences in recent demographic trends between Mission churches and Independent or so-called 'Spirit-type' churches. It is argued that the latter, with more restrictive norms on alcohol consumption and extra-marital relationships, may limit the spread of HIV and thereby reduce mortality among church members. These findings support the view that contrasting HIV epidemics seen between sub-Saharan African sub-populations can at least partly be explained by differences in sexual behaviours. It might also be the case that 'Spirit-type' churches grow in popularity in the future as the severe consequences of the AIDS epidemic become more apparent. Their appeal seems to lie in the parallels they provide with traditional custom, their strict moral codes, and the reassurances they offer in times of change - characteristics which make them attractive in the midst of the epidemic. HIV/AIDS might thus become an important influence in the future evolution of churches and religious teaching in Zimbabwe.

Jones, P. (2004) 'When 'development' devastates: donor discourses, access to HIV/AIDS treatment in Africa and rethinking the landscape of development', *Third World Quarterly* **25** , pp. 385-404.

This article takes the view that if globalisation can be seen as shaking the landscape of development, then, at least in certain regions of the world, HIV/AIDS is at its epicentre. Inspite of the by now well documented and visible impact of the pandemic, however, Western donor policies on HIV/AIDS are characterized by pervasive medical neglect and a strong preference for prevention programmes over treatment. The paper explains those policies - using the UK Department for International Development and the Norwegian Agency for Development Co-operation as illustrations - as framed by certain representations of 'Africa' in the wider Western discourse. Those representations and the construction of North-South relations more generally are described as being premised upon representations of the

North as the privileged centre of knowledge, authority and power. The paper argues for a comprehensive reconstruction of the project of development. In relation to HIV/AIDS policies this is suggested to mean the foregrounding of a human right to health as including, critically, the promotion of treatment within a genuine 'prevention-care-treatment' policy continuum.

Kalipeni, E., S. **Craddock**, J. **Oppong** and J. **Gosh** (eds.) (2004) *HIV and AIDS in Africa. Beyond Epidemiology*. Oxford: Blackwell Publishing.

This book sets out to be an intervention into the predominant understanding of AIDS in Africa based on biomedical models of individual risk and rational behavioural change at a time when their lack of success in intervening into the epidemic has become evident. It aims to uncover the various ways in which AIDS is embedded within social, economic, cultural, political and ideological contexts. AIDS is thus understood as deeply rooted in historical antecedents, geopolitical relations, and global financial configurations, as well as in government policies, local institutions and cultural politics. The five different parts of the book reflect this range of issues: Part one deals with historical investigations into the impact of colonialism on African economies and social practices as pivotal to understanding regional patterns of HIV transmission today. Part two discusses the pattern of the spread of HIV/AIDS in Africa and its direction of change over the last 20 years, while part three focuses on social issues around HIV/AIDS, in concrete on the three areas of gendered vulnerabilities, sexualities and identities, and the effects of poverty, war and migration on HIV transmission and its interpretation. Part four focuses on research methods, research agendas and ethical questions, and part five centres on impact and wider repercussions of the pandemic in Africa. Though the contributors vary in their conceptual approaches to understanding AIDS, they employ for the most part variations of a 'cultural political economy of vulnerability framework' that reflects an understanding of AIDS as resulting from material, symbolic, and discursive forces effectively constraining the opportunities and choices available to individuals, and potentially creating conditions of vulnerability for large sectors of different populations. As such, the book is a good starting point for a more holistic understanding of HIV/AIDS and a valuable contribution to the wider debate on HIV/AIDS as a human development issue (see also Brown, 2004; Lurie et al., 2004; Schoepf, 2004; and Zulu et al., 2004 for individual chapters).

Loewenson, R. and A. **Whiteside** (2001) 'HIV/AIDS. Implications for Poverty Reduction'. Background paper prepared for the United Nations Development Programme for the UN General Assembly Special Session on HIV/AIDS, 25-27 June 2001, New York.

This paper looks at HIV/AIDS in relation to internationally adopted poverty reduction strategies with a special focus on the MDGs. It is argued that the response to the epidemic has thus far focused on containment and prevention of new infections through advocacy, information and education campaigns, condom distribution and similar interventions, coupled with a focus on care and treatment. In doing so, this response has ignored the 'bigger picture' of the epidemic's implications for human development in general and poverty reduction in particular. Compounding this shortcoming, national and global development targets have been formulated without taking the added challenges resulting from sharp increases in AIDS-related adult mortality rates into account. This argument is exemplified by a table discussing some of the MDGs and the impact of AIDS on progress towards those goals. The paper continues - after having discussed the multi-faceted socio-economic impact of the epidemic - by identifying and discussing five priorities for action in coping with this impact: the prevention of the collapse of essential services; adaptation of poverty reduction efforts in the light of the respective epidemics within each geographical setting; protection of educational achievements; mitigation of the impact on labour productivity and supply; and the promotion of opportunities for women. The paper ends by emphasizing the crucial role of national leadership combined with international support in addressing the developmental impact of the epidemic.

Mather, D., C. **Donovan**, T. **Jayne**, M. **Weber**, E. **Mazhangara**, L. **Bailey**, K. **Yoo**, T. **Yamano** and E. **Mghenyi** (2004b) *A Cross-Country Analysis of Household Responses to Adult Mortality in Rural sub-Saharan Africa: Implications for HIV/AIDS Mitigation and Rural Development*

Policies. Michigan: Michigan State University, Department of Agricultural Economics.

This paper synthesizes across the results of a set of country studies on the effects of prime-age adult mortality on rural households. Countries covered are Kenya, Malawi, Mozambique, Rwanda and Zambia (see also Donovan et al., 2003; Mather et al., 2004a) . Each study is based on large representative rural household surveys. While survey instruments in each country differed to some extent, in each survey information was collected that links household and individual economic attributes with health and mortality status. Information collected from each setting thus includes data on agricultural and livestock production and sales, off-farm activities, land use, income and livelihood sources, and available services, as well as socioeconomic characteristics of each current household member and information with regard to household members who have either died or departed. Among the main findings are the following: Incidence of prime-age adult mortality due to illness is a reasonably accurate way to identify households that are most likely affected by HIV/AIDS-related mortality. In contrast to more general assumptions, in four out of the five countries the majority of diseased prime-age adults were not the household heads or spouses and thus not the primary providers for the household. Again in contrast to widely held beliefs, households that experienced prime-age adult death did not necessarily have less prime-adult labour available, nor did the average affected household have necessarily less land cultivated or experienced an overall negative effect on crop production. More generally it was found that the gender and household position of the diseased, combined with the initial assets level, appears to strongly condition the overall effect of prime-age adult death on the household, with for example poorer households headed by widows likely to be in the most precarious situation. These findings lead to a questioning of the widely held assumption that HIV/AIDS mitigation policy should prioritize agricultural labour-saving technologies and food aid targeted to affected households. It might indeed be more important to address issues such as improved land and tenure security for women; the gender bias in agricultural production and marketing knowledge as well as in cash crop and non-farm opportunities; and to invest in labour-saving technologies for domestic tasks such as food processing and water or fuel gathering. Overall the paper argues that HIV/AIDS mitigation policies need to be tied to agricultural and rural economic development policies that redress constraints to pro-poor and gender-sensitive economic growth.

Msiska, R. (2002) *Conceptual Shifts for Sound Planning: Towards an Integrated Approach to HIV/AIDS and Poverty*. Pretoria: UNDP Regional Project on HIV and Development.
http://www.sarpn.org.za/documents/d0000130/Conseptual_shifts_for_sound_plannig.pdf, accessed 18 April 2005.

This paper is based on the assumption, based on global trends, that the HIV/AIDS pandemic is at an early stage and its long-term evolution is still far from clear. What is clear, however, is that the pandemic poses one of the most critical development challenges for sub-Saharan Africa. As one of the reasons why sub-Saharan Africa is particularly vulnerable to HIV/AIDS, the high levels of poverty in many parts of the continent are singled out. Because HIV/AIDS in sub-Saharan Africa is predominately spread through heterosexual encounters, the paper as a starting point reviews what is known about sexual behaviour, placing such behaviour within the overall social, political, economic and technological environment. In a next step, poverty as understood in the context of the paper is conceptualized. The following sections then explore in some detail the relationship between poverty and HIV/AIDS and vice versa, providing a useful overview of the relevant issues in question at individual, household and community level and at all stages of HIV and AIDS. The paper ends with proposing some models for an integrated response to poverty and HIV/AIDS, looking at how HIV/AIDS could be mainstreamed into poverty reduction strategies from a prevention as well as an impact perspective.

Müller, T. (2005b) 'Responding to the HIV/AIDS epidemic. Lessons from the case of Eritrea', *Progress in Development Studies* **5**, pp. 199-212.

This paper discusses the political response to HIV/AIDS in Eritrea, a country where the epidemic appears to have stabilized at an average prevalence rate of around three percent. It shows that Eritrea has mobilized an effective multisectoral response to cope with the epidemic and its impact under conditions of full-scale war followed by a still fragile post-conflict situation, compounded by recurring drought and economic decline. As one key factor for successful policy action the commitment of a centralised government with the capacity to implement its decisions and mobilize other stakeholders is identified. Another important factor might be the high level of social cohesion prevalent within Eritrean society.

Over, M. (1992) *The Macroeconomic Impact of AIDS in sub-Saharan Africa*. Washington DC: World Bank.

This paper estimates the macroeconomic impact of AIDS on economies in sub-Saharan Africa by projecting the growth trajectories of 30 countries with and without the AIDS epidemic over the period 1990-2025. It is shown that if the only effect of AIDS were to reduce the population growth rate, the growth rate of per capita income would increase in any plausible economic model. The paper then asks whether the specific characteristics of the AIDS epidemic would be sufficient to reverse this prediction, so that per capita income growth would turn out to be negative. The characteristics examined are the effect of the epidemic on savings and the distribution of the epidemic by socio-economic class, which is called the 'socio-economic gradient' of the epidemic. For the assumptions regarded as most plausible concerning this 'socio-economic gradient' the net effect of the AIDS epidemic on the growth of per capita income is a reduction of about a third of a percentage point in the ten countries with the most advanced epidemics - in a continent struggling to escape negative growth of per capita income a substantial additional burden. The paper then outlines some possible policy implications: If for example the maximisation of per capita economic growth were the only objective, the results argue for targeting prevention efforts at the more highly educated members of society. But, it is acknowledged, there are other considerations which must be weighed in targeting prevention efforts, not least equity considerations. Ultimately, it is argued, policy guidance can only come from microeconomic studies that investigate the determinants of the impact's magnitude on surviving household members and the effectiveness of alternative approaches towards impact mitigation.

Putzel, J. (2003) *Institutionalising an Emergency Response: HIV/AIDS and Governance in Uganda and Senegal*. London: Department for International Development (DFID).

This report examines the impact of governance on controlling HIV/AIDS, taking the examples of Uganda and Senegal. Four central aspects of political leadership are identified that have made Uganda and Senegal - two very different countries with two very different epidemics - engage with the epidemic. These are a) an incentive structure in which leaders had little to lose and everything to gain from engaging in the fight against HIV/AIDS; b) leaders came to act on the basis of medical and scientific evidence; c) it became illegitimate for anyone to occupy a position of government without fully committing to the fight against AIDS; d) central leaders were pivotal to the mobilisation of social organisations. More generally, a tension between principles of democracy and respect for individual rights on the one hand, and imperatives of securing public health on the other is discussed. It is advocated to consider more compulsory measures where conditions warrant and capacity exists to engage in those constructively. In addition, the transformation of economic activity in terms of modernisation and development has often brought with it displacement, labour migrations and long-distance trading, all factors which possibly contribute to the spread of HIV/AIDS. The AIDS crisis thus makes it necessary to rethink strategies of economic change, something that has not seriously begun. Overall, the tensions involved in responding to the AIDS crisis make it necessary to look at governance analytically and politically, not merely as a checklist of functions and best practices. While on the one hand emergency action is called for, the nature of the emergency is long-term, thus demanding an institutionalised emergency response.

Rugalema, G. (2000) 'Coping or Struggling? A Journey into the Impact of HIV/AIDS in Southern Africa', *Review of African Political Economy (ROAPE)* **86**, pp. 537-545.

The article questions the wisdom of employing the notion of coping strategies to analyse the effects of morbidity and mortality associated with HIV/AIDS in rural Africa. It is argued that in areas hard hit by AIDS the concept of coping strategies is of limited value in explaining household experiences and may in fact serve to divert policy-makers from the enormity of the emergency. To say that households are coping implies they are at the very least persevering. Research, however, has shown that adult mortality in a considerable number of cases results in household dissolution, a clear indication of a failure to cope. The conceptual framework built around the notion of coping is derived from famine survival strategies of rural households. Such strategies might be ill suited to analyse household responses to morbidity and mortality associated with HIV/AIDS.

Stillwaggon, E. (2000) 'HIV Transmission in Latin America: Comparison with Africa and Policy Implications', *The South African Journal of Economics* **68**, pp. 985-1011.

The starting point of this article is that the global HIV/AIDS pandemic has developed under diverse socio-economic conditions leading to variations in the mode and rate of transmission between countries, regions and continents. It draws on lessons from sub-Saharan Africa in examining some of the economic and biomedical determinants of HIV transmission in Latin America and the Caribbean where, it is argued, such factors have been largely overlooked because AIDS policy has been framed narrowly in behavioural terms that had proved useful in guiding policy in the United States and Europe. The paper shows that in much of Latin America and the Caribbean it have increasingly been countries with higher levels of poverty, greater inequality, and lower levels of nutrition and access to health care that have had higher incidences of HIV. More generally, it is concluded that in the developing world - while behaviour-modification programmes can be useful - those are no substitutes for economic policies that promote equitable development, and social policies that provide preventive and curative care.

Takyi, B. (2003) 'Religion and women's health in Ghana: insights into HIV/AIDS preventive and protective behaviour', *Social Science & Medicine* **56**, pp. 1221-1234.

The article analyses the interrelationship between religion and AIDS behaviour in Ghana. At the time of writing the AIDS epidemic in Ghana was at an early stage. At the same time religious activities in Ghana are very pronounced. The hypothesis behind studying religion and sexual behaviour assumes that religion may foster social capital networks through which the diffusion of HIV/AIDS information is bound to occur. In Ghana it are in particular women who spend considerable time in faith- and church-based interactions. Findings, based on data from the 1998 Ghana Demographic Health Survey, indicate that religious affiliation has indeed a significant effect on knowledge of AIDS among Ghanaian women. The study did not, however, find religious affiliation to be associated with changes towards protective behaviour.

UNAIDS (2005) *AIDS in Africa: Three scenarios to 2025.* Geneva: UNAIDS.

The overall aim of this project has been to explore how seemingly disconnected events - such as patterns of global trade, the education of women and girls, terrorist attacks on the other side of the world, the rise of certain political regimes - can influence the course of the HIV/AIDS pandemic. Three possible scenarios are presented on how Africa may look twenty years from now, in 2025. The focus is on the factors that drive Africa's and the world's response to the HIV/AIDS pandemic, and on what kind of future there will be for the coming generations of Africans. Those scenarios are narrated under the headlines 'Tough Choices', 'Traps and Legacies: The Whirlpool', and 'Times of Transition: Africa overcomes'. They are not meant as predictions, but as plausible stories about the future, depending on what action is or is not taken today. The key message of 'Tough Choices' is that there is much Africa can do on its own in an overall context in which attitudes and practices of the rest of the world towards Africa are unlikely to change. This scenario shows that with leadership and community mobilization effective HIV/AIDS responses are possible even without huge outlays of resources on stand-alone programming. The scenario thus ends with declining HIV incidence (even though the absolute number of PLWHA remains the same as at the beginning due to population momentum) as long-term investments in social, economic and human capital over two decades begin to pay dividend. The essential message from 'Traps and Legacies' is that it will be difficult to make a difference to the pandemic if HIV/AIDS is viewed in isolation from its root social, economic and political context. It is a story of good intentions thwarted by an underlying development malaise that remains unchanged. In this scenario the African continent is gripped in a downward spiral of disunity, denial and stigma, contested knowledge, wasted resources and competing sources of power and authority. Population growth in this scenario will translate existing rates of incidence and prevalence into a doubling of the number of PLWHA between now and 2025. Finally, 'Times of Transition' describes a scenario in which Africa and the rest of the world together approach the issues of health, development, trade, security and international relations, a scenario in which the HIV/AIDS pandemic magnifies a wider crisis and acts as a catalyst for action, by states as well as by civil society. The transitions require sustained social investment and fundamental changes in the way in which donors provide aid and governments deal with it - so that aid promotes sovereignty but does not undermine national autonomy or promote dependency. 'Times of Transition' is based on a new understanding of solidarity and citizenship, globally and locally. The scenario suggests that if these transitions can be made within a generation they can dramatically reduce the number of PLWHA and fundamentally alter the future course of Africa and the world in the 21st century.

United Nations (2004) *The Impact of AIDS*. New York: UN, Department of Economic and Social Affairs, Population Division.

This report documents the wide-ranging impacts of HIV/AIDS on individuals, families and nations based on a review of existing literature. It consists of two parts. Part one discusses in nine different chapters all dimensions of HIV/AIDS impact. The first chapter considers data, sources and methods for studying impact. The second chapter looks at demographic changes caused by the pandemic in particular in relation to the most severely affected countries. It is followed by a chapter on impact on families and households. Chapter four and five address impact on the production sector of the economy, namely firms and agriculture. The next two chapters discuss impact on the education and health sector respectively, followed by a chapter discussing impact on national economic growth. In chapter nine some conclusions are discussed. The second part consists of summaries of selected studies on HIV/AIDS impact already referred to in the earlier chapters. The report thus provides a general introduction into the different aspects of HIV/AIDS impact from where more specialised interests can then be pursued. Its main recommendation is for all countries to develop and implement national strategies to promote the delivery of comprehensive prevention, treatment, care, and support to those living with or being affected by HIV/AIDS.

Whiteside, A. (2002) 'Poverty and HIV/AIDS in Africa', *Third World Quarterly* **23**, pp. 313-332.

The article looks at HIV/AIDS as the major threat to development, economic growth and poverty alleviation in sub-Saharan Africa. It starts by describing the epidemic, explaining its importance and what makes it different from other development threats. It then explores how the poverty-epidemic cycle works, whereby poverty increases the spread of HIV and AIDS increases poverty. Furthermore, it is criticized that the potential impact of HIV/AIDS on households and societies is not included in the UN's Millennium Development Targets, thus ignoring the fact that the epidemic might put these targets into jeopardy. For selected targets the impact of HIV/AIDS on progress towards that target as well as steps to be taken to achieve it within a context of HIV/AIDS are outlined. Furthermore, areas into which future research would be helpful are identified. These include: the relationship between inequality and communicable disease in general and HIV/AIDS in particular; the effect of the epidemic on relational goods, public goods and issues of social reproduction. Overall, the article raises similar points as are argued in Loewenson and Whiteside (2001) and Barnett and Whiteside (2002).

Additional sources

Ainsworth, M. and I. Semali (1998) 'Who is most likely to die of AIDS? Socioeconomic correlates of adult deaths in Kagera Region, Tanzania', in M. Ainsworth, L. Fransen and M. Over (eds.) *Confronting AIDS: Evidence from the Developing World, selected background papers for the World Bank Policy Research Report Confronting AIDS: Public Priorities in a Global Epidemic*, pp. 95-109. Luxembourg: Office for Official Publications of the European Commission.

Allison, E. and J. Seeley (2004) 'HIV and AIDS among fisherfolk: a threat to 'responsible fisheries'?', *Fish and Fisheries* **5**, pp. 215-234.

Ayieko, M. (1997) *From Single Parents to Children-Headed Households: The Case of Children Orphaned by AIDS in Kisumu and Siaya Districts*. HIV and Development Programme, Study Paper No. **7**. New York: UNDP.

Barnett, T. (2003) 'HIV/AIDS, Human Development and the Coming Epidemic in the Balkans, Baltic, Russian Federation and the CIS', in Agence Nationale de Recherches sur le SIDA (ANRS) (ed.) *Economics of AIDS and Access to HIV/AIDS Care in Developing Countries. Issues and Challenges*, pp. 413-433. Paris: ANRS.

Barnett, T. (2004) 'HIV and serious anthropology', *Anthropology Today* **20**, pp. 2-3.

Barnett, T. and P. Blaikie (1992) *AIDS in Africa. Its present and future impact*. London: Belhaven Press.

Barnett, T., J. Tumushabe, G. Bantebya, R. Ssebuliba, J. Ngasongwa, D. Kapinga, M. Ndelike, M. Drinkwater, G. Mitti and M. Haslwimmer (1995) 'The Social and Economic Impact of HIV/AIDS on Farming Systems and Livelihoods in Rural Africa: Some Experience and Lessons from Uganda, Tanzania and Zambia', *Journal of International Development* **7**, pp. 163-176.

Barnett, T. and A. Whiteside (1999a) 'HIV/AIDS in Africa: Implications for "development" and major policy implications'. Paper presented at the Fourth SCUSA Inter-University Colloquium, 5-8 September 1999, University of East Anglia, Norwich.

Barnett, T. and A. Whiteside (1999b) 'HIV/AIDS and Development: Case Studies and a Conceptual Framework', *The European Journal of Development Research* **11**, pp. 200-234.

Bell, C., S. Devarajan and H. Gersbach (2003) *The Long-run Economic Costs of AIDS: Theory and an Application to South Africa*. Washington DC: World Bank.

Bennell, P., K. Hyde and N. Swainson (2002) *The impact of the HIV/AIDS epidemic on the education sector in sub-Saharan Africa. A synthesis of the findings and recommendations of three country studies*. Sussex: Centre for International Education, University of Sussex.

Björkman, H. (2002) *HIV/AIDS and Poverty Reduction Strategies.* New York: UNDP.

Bloom, D. and A. Mahal (1997) 'Does the AIDS epidemic threaten economic growth?', *Journal of Econometrics* **77**, pp. 105-124.

Bollinger, L., J. Stover and M. Palamuleni (2000) *The Economic Impact of AIDS in Malawi.* Washington DC: Futures Group International.

Bollinger, L., J. Stover and P. Riwa (1999) *The Economic Impact of AIDS in Tanzania.* Washington DC: Futures Group International.

Booysen, F. (2003) 'Poverty Dynamics and HIV/AIDS-related morbidity and mortality in South Africa'. Paper presented at the Scientific Meeting on Empirical Evidence for the Demographic and Socio-Economic Impact of AIDS, 26-28 March 2003, University of Natal, Durban, South Africa.

Brown, L. (2004) 'Economic Growth Rates in Africa: The Potential Impact of HIV/AIDS', in E. Kalipeni, S. Craddock, J. Oppong and J. Gosh (eds.) *HIV and AIDS in Africa. Beyond Epidemiology*, pp. 291-303. Oxford: Blackwell Publishing.

Brown, L., P. Webb and L. Haddad (1994) 'The role of labour in household food security: implications of AIDS in Africa', *Food Policy* **19**, pp. 568-573.

Bujra, J. (2004) 'AIDS as a Crisis in Social Reproduction', *Review of African Political Economy* **102**, pp. 631-638.

Cuddington, J. (1993) 'Further Results on the Macroeconomic Effects of AIDS: The Dualistic, Labour-Surplus Economy', *The World Bank Economic Review* **7**, pp. 403-417.

Cuddington, J. and J. Hancock (1995) 'The Macroeconomic Impact of AIDS in Malawi: a Dualistic, Labour Surplus Economy', *Journal of African Economies* **4**, pp. 1-28.

de Cock, K., D. Mbori-Ngacha and E. Marum (2002) 'Shadow on the continent: public health and HIV/AIDS in Africa in the 21st century', *The Lancet* **360**, pp. 67-72.

Donovan, C., L. Bailey, E. Mpyisi and M. Weber (2003) *Prime-Age Adult Morbidity and Mortality in Rural Rwanda: Effects on Household Income, Agricultural Production, and Food Security Strategies.* Kigali, Rwanda: Ministry of Agriculture, Livestock, and Forestry.

Fredland, R. (1998) 'AIDS and development: an inverse correlation?', *The Journal of Modern African Studies* **36**, pp. 547-568.

Gerald, K. (2004) Transhumance as a Factor in the HIV/AIDS Epidemic in the Pastoral Communities of sub-Saharan Africa. MSc Thesis in Tropical Animal Production, Deventer, Larenstein University.

Gillespie, S. (1989) 'Potential Impact of AIDS on farming systems. A case study from Rwanda', *Land Use Policy* **6**, pp. 301-312.

Gillespie, S., L. Haddad and R. Jackson (2001) 'HIV/AIDS, Food and Nutrition Security: Impacts and Actions'.

http://www.fantaproject.org/downloads/pdfs/IFPRI2001_hivaids.pdf, accessed 18 April 2005.

Glynn, J., M. Caraël, A. Buvé, S. Anagonou, L. Zekeng, M. Kahindo and R. Musonda (2004) 'Does increased general schooling protect against HIV infection? A study in four African cities', *Tropical Medicine and International Health* **9**, pp. 4-14.

Gray, P. (2004) 'HIV and Islam: is HIV prevalence lower among Muslims?', *Social Science & Medicine* **58**, pp. 1751-1756.

Gregson, S., H. Waddell and S. Chandiwana (2001) 'School education and HIV control in sub-Saharan Africa: From discord to harmony?', *Journal of International Development* **13**, pp. 467-485.

Hallman, K. (2004) *Socioeconomic Disadvantage and Unsafe Sexual Behaviours Among Young Women and Men in South Africa*. Policy Research Division Working paper No. **190**. New York: Population Council.

International Organisation for Migration (IOM) (2003) *Mobility and HIV/AIDS in Southern Africa: A field study in South Africa, Zimbabwe and Mozambique*. Geneva: IOM.

Kipp, W., P. Kabwa, A. Verbeck, P. Fischer, P. Eggert and D. Büttner (1995) 'Prevalence and risk factors of HIV-1 infection in three parishes in western Uganda', *Trop. Med. Parasitol.* **46**, pp. 141-146.

Klouda, T. (1995) 'Responding to AIDS: Are There *Any* Appropriate Development and Health Policies?', *Journal of International Development* **7**, pp. 467-487.

Krieger, N. (2001) 'Theories for social epidemiology in the 21st century: an ecosocial perspective', *International Journal of Epidemiology* **30**, pp. 668-677.

Loewenson, R. and A. Whiteside (1997) *Social and Economic Issues of HIV/AIDS in Southern Africa*. A Consultancy Report. Harare: Southern Africa AIDS Information Dissemination Service (SAfAIDS).

Love, R. (2004) 'HIV/AIDS in Africa: Links, Livelihoods and Legacies', *Review of African Political Economy* **102**, pp. 639-648.

Low-Beer, D. and R. Stoneburner (2003) 'Behaviour and communication change in reducing HIV: is Uganda unique?', *African Journal of AIDS research* **2**, pp. 9-21.

Lurie, P., P. Hintzen and R. Lowe (2004) 'Socioeconomic Obstacles to HIV Prevention and Treatment in Developing Countries: The Roles of the International Monetary Fund and the World Bank', in E. Kalipeni, S. Craddock, J. Oppong and J. Gosh (eds.) *HIV and AIDS in Africa. Beyond Epidemiology*, pp. 204-212. Oxford: Blackwell Publishing.

Mather, D., H. Marrule, C. Donovan, M. Weber and A. Alage (2004a) *Analysis of Adult Mortality Within Rural Households in Mozambique and Implications for Policy*. Maputo, Mozambique: Ministry of Agriculture and Rural Development.

Maxwell, J. (2003) 'What is Social Cohesion, and Why Do We Care?'. Montreal: Canadian Policy Research Networks.

Morton, J. (2003) 'Conceptualising the links between HIV/AIDS and pastoralist livelihoods'. Paper presented at the Annual Conference of the Development Studies Association, 10 - 12 September 2003, Glasgow.

Muelder, A. (2004) 'Implications of HIV/AIDS for Pro-Poor Agricultural Growth'. Paper presented in the session on Chronic Poverty in the POVNET Agriculture Helsinki Workshop, 17-18 June 2004, Helsinki.

Müller, T. (2004a) *HIV/AIDS and agriculture in sub-Saharan Africa. Impact on farming systems, agricultural practices and rural livelihoods - an overview and annotated bibliography.* Wageningen: Wageningen Academic Publishers.

Müller, T. (2004b) 'Responding to the HIV/AIDS Epidemics: Lessons from successful interventions'. Paper presented at the Conference Where Science Meets Society, 23 April 2004, Wageningen University and Research Centre.

Müller, T. (2005a) *HIV/AIDS, gender and rural livelihoods in sub-Saharan Africa. An overview and annotated bibliography.* Wageningen: Wageningen Academic Publishers.

Mushati, P., S. Gregson, M. Mlilo, C. Zvidzai and C. Nyamukapa (2003) 'Adult mortality and erosion of household viability in AIDS-afflicted towns, estates and villages in eastern Zimbabwe'. Paper presented at the Scientific Meeting on Empirical Evidence for the Demographic and Socio-Economic Impact of AIDS, 26-28 March 2003, University of Natal, Durban, South Africa.

Ngom, P. and S. Clark (2003) 'Adult Mortality in the Era of HIV/AIDS: Sub-Saharan Africa'. Paper presented at the Workshop on HIV/AIDS and adult mortality in developing countries, Population Division, Department of Economic and Social Affairs, United Nations Secretariat, 8-13 September 2003, New York.

Over, M. (1998) 'The effects of societal variables on urban rates of HIV infection in developing countries: An exploratory analysis', in M. Ainsworth, L. Fransen and M. Over (eds.) *Confronting AIDS: Evidence from the Developing World, selected background papers for the World Bank Policy Research Report Confronting AIDS: Public Priorities in a Global Epidemic*, pp. 39-51. Luxembourg: Office for Official Publications of the European Commission.

Parker, R., D. Easton and C. Klein (2000) 'Structural barriers and facilitators in HIV prevention: a review of international research', *AIDS* **14**, pp. S22-S32.

Piot, P. (2005) 'Why AIDS is exceptional', speech given at the London School of Economics on 8 February 2005.

Price-Smith, A. and J. Daly (2004) *Downward Spiral. HIV/AIDS, State Capacity, and Political Conflict in Zimbabwe.* Washington DC: United States Institute of Peace.

Putzel, J. (2004) 'The Politics of Action on AIDS: A Case Study of Uganda', *Public Administration and Development* **24**, pp. 19-30.

Rosen, S. and J. Simon (2002) *Shifting the Burden of HIV/AIDS*. Health and Development Discussion Paper No. **1**. Boston: Centre for International Health, Boston University, School of Public Health.

Roth, E., E. Fratkin, A. Eastman and L. Nathan (1999) 'Knowledge of AIDS Among Ariaal Pastoralists of Northern Kenya', *Nomadic Peoples* **3**, pp. 161-175.

Schoepf, B. (2004) 'AIDS, History, and Struggles over Meaning', in E. Kalipeni, S. Craddock, J. Oppong and J. Gosh (eds.) *HIV and AIDS in Africa. Beyond Epidemiology*, pp. 15-28. Oxford: Blackwell Publishing.

Schoepf, B. (2003) 'Uganda: Lessons for AIDS Control in Africa', *Review of African Political Economy* **98**, pp. 553-572.

Shah, M., N. Osborne, T. Mbilizi and G. Vilili (2002) *Impact of HIV/AIDS on Agricultural Productivity and Rural Livelihoods in the Central Region of Malawi*. Lilongwe: CARE International Malawi.

Stover, J. (1998) 'The future demographic impact of AIDS: What do we know?', in M. Ainsworth, L. Fransen and M. Over (eds.) *Confronting AIDS: Evidence from the Developing World, selected background papers for the World Bank Policy Research Report Confronting AIDS: Public Priorities in a Global Epidemic*, pp. 11-38. Luxembourg: Office for Official Publications of the European Commission.

Tanzarn, N. and C. Bishop-Sambrook (2003) *The Dynamics of HIV/AIDS in Small-Scale Fishing Communities in Uganda*. Rome: United Nations Food and Agricultural Organisation (FAO).

The Economist (17 April 2004) 'Special Report: AIDS in India', pp. 21-23.

UNAIDS (2004) *2004 Report on the global AIDS epidemic*. Geneva: UNAIDS.

UNAIDS/WHO (2004) *AIDS epidemic update December 2004*. Geneva: UNAIDS/WHO.

United Nations Development Programme (UNDP) (2004) *HIV/AIDS in Eastern Europe and the Commonwealth of Independent States. Reversing the Epidemic. Facts and Policy Options*. Bratislava: UNDP.

White, J. and E. Robinson (2000) *HIV/AIDS and Rural Livelihoods in Sub-Saharan Africa*. Policy Series **6**. Greenwich: Natural Resources Institute, University of Greenwich.

Whiteside, A., T. Barnett, G. George and A. van Niekerk (2003) 'Through a glass, darkly: data and uncertainty in the AIDS debate', *Developing World Bioethics* **3**, pp. 49-76.

Willan, S. (2004) 'Briefing: Recent Changes in the South African Government's HIV/AIDS policy and its implementations', *African Affairs* **103**, pp. 109-117.

Worst, P. and C. Arndt (2004) 'HIV/AIDS and Labour Force Upgrading in Tanzania', *World Development* **32**, pp. 1831-1847.

Yamano, T. and T. Jayne (2004) 'Measuring the Impacts of Working-Age Adult Mortality on Small-Scale Farm Households in Kenya', *World Development* **32**, pp. 91-119.

Zhang, H. (2004) 'The Gathering Storm: AIDS Policy in China', *Journal of International Development* **16**, pp. 1155-1168.

Zulu, E., F. Dodoo and A. Ezeh (2004) 'Urbanization, Poverty, and Sex: Roots of Risky Sexual Behaviours in Slum Settlements in Nairobi, Kenya', in E. Kalipeni, S. Craddock, J. Oppong and J. Gosh (eds.) *HIV and AIDS in Africa. Beyond Epidemiology*, pp. 167-174. Oxford: Blackwell Publishing.

2. HIV/AIDS mitigation through agricultural interventions and beyond

Agence Nationale de Recherches sur le SIDA (ANRS) (2003) *Economics of AIDS and Access to HIV/AIDS Care in Developing Countries. Issues and Challenges.* Paris: ANRS.

This book is first and foremost a contribution to the debate on expanding access to HIV/AIDS treatment in developing countries. Part one of the book focuses on 'patents, generic drugs and the market for antiretrovirals', or on the conflictual interactions between drugs-related intellectual property rights, particularly in relation to the Trade-Related Aspects of Intellectual Property Rights (TRIPS) agreement signed in 1994, and access to treatment. The second part of the book deals with AIDS impact and the expansion of effective therapeutic strategies. All its papers present evidence to support the idea that scaling up access to ART and other effective treatments for HIV/AIDS can be a rational economic choice for developing countries. In addition the conditions to be met and the policies to be implemented in order to maximize the benefits from such access are discussed. The underlying message here is that denying expanded access to ART is not only unethical and detrimental to public health, it is also bad economy policy (see also Coriat et al., 2003; Eholie et al., 2003; Freedberg & Yazdanpanah, 2003; Moatti et al., 2003b; and Orsi et al., 2003, for specific parts of this publication).

Aliber, M., C. **Walker**, M. **Machera**, P. **Kamau**, C. **Omondi** and K. **Kanyinga** (2004) *The Impact of HIV/AIDS on Land Rights. Case Studies from Kenya*. Cape Town: Human Sciences Research Council (HSRC) Publishers.

This is the report of an in-depth investigation into the link between HIV/AIDS and land tenure in three rural sites in Kenya conducted in 2002. The three sites are located in Embu, Thika and Bondo districts, in Eastern, Central and Nyanza Provinces respectively. Research methods involved a combination of participatory research techniques, household surveys, and in-depth person-to-person interviews, and attempted to distinguish the role of HIV/AIDS in aggravating tenure insecurity from other factors. Although falling short of a nationally representative sample, the findings allow for some cross-regional and cross-cultural comparisons. The overarching finding confirms conclusions from earlier studies that HIV/AIDS can undermine tenure security of some community members, but also shows that such threats do not necessarily result in actual loss of tenure status. The study also reports little evidence of distress sales of land as a consequence of HIV/AIDS, and far fewer examples of dispossession of widows' or orphans' land rights than the general literature and anecdotal accounts had suggested. Overall, also in relation to groups generally regarded as vulnerable such as widows, the study finds that a link between HIV/AIDS and land tenure loss is neither omnipresent nor the norm. It is thus cautioned against focusing predominately on HIV/AIDS as a threat to tenure security. There are many other pressures on land rights - the most prominent being poverty and unequal gender relations - which impact on both AIDS afflicted, AIDS affected and non-affected households. The concrete impact of HIV/AIDS on land rights is to a great degree context specific, depending on land pressure, 'cultural' reactions to HIV/AIDS including denial or stigma, and the status of women. One implication of those findings - given the fact that tenure insecurity is experienced by many households irrespective of their particular exposure to AIDS - is that one should be wary of giving preference to AIDS afflicted households when designing protection measures.

Barnett, T. and R. **Grellier** (2003) *Mitigation of the Impact of HIV/AIDS on Rural Livelihoods Through Low-Labour Input Agriculture and Related Activities*. Norwich: Overseas Development Group.

This consultancy report addresses the following issues: the kind of impact the HIV/AIDS pandemic has on rural livelihoods, with a focus on field-based subsistence agriculture in sub-Saharan Africa (the focus of most of the available literature); evidence of indigenous responses within HIV/AIDS affected rural communities; and the potential of labour economising technologies to mitigate HIV/AIDS impact in such communities. The first section of the report address those issues in discussing the findings from available studies (published as well as electronically available materials). The second part is based on structured fieldwork conducted in Uganda, Tanzania, Malawi and Zambia, with some additional reference to data from Mozambique and Nigeria. This fieldwork consists mainly of semi-structured interviews with representatives of organisations working with or supporting others involved in labour economising technologies and include Ministry of Agriculture officials and extension workers, as well as chief executives of NGOs and community-based organisations. Findings include the following: HIV/AIDS impact on rural livelihoods has been widely evident in central, eastern and southern Africa. The normal response to this impact has been a downshifting of the rural economy to a survival mode combined with a reallocation of labour. In such an environment, the only truly labour economising technology is seen in the provision of ARVs. The report ends with outlining eleven policy options, ranging from option number one, to do nothing, to option number eleven, called de 'deluxe' option: This would involve the introduction of ARVs together with social protection mechanisms and labour economising technologies in a manner that people could join the latter according to their own capabilities, needs and priorities (what is called the 'stairway approach'). It is argued that only this last option would give labour economising technologies a chance to work (as people on ARVs remain capable of being economically and socially active members of their communities), while preventing (through social protection mechanisms and 'stairway' introduction) people to become socially excluded or face even greater destitution if such technologies do not live up to their initial promises.

Bishop-Sambrook, C. (2003b) *Labour Saving Technologies and Practices for Farming and Household Activities in Eastern and Southern Africa. Labour Constraints and the Impact of HIV/AIDS on Rural Livelihoods in Bondo and Busia Districts, Western Kenya*. Rome: International Fund for Agricultural Development (IFAD) and the United Nations Food and Agricultural Organisation (FAO).

The starting point for this report is the assumption that human and draught power will continue to be the main source of farm power in the foreseeable future, with hand power being critical within the production process, both in terms of availability and productivity (it is estimated that 65 percent of land in sub-Saharan Africa is prepared by hand power). Both those variables, however, are compromised through poor nutrition; illness (often AIDS-induced) and death; competing claims on time for labour intensive household tasks; and the drift away from the land in search of alternatives to subsistence agriculture. Within this context, the purpose of a field study on which this report is based was threefold: to identify labour/power shortages in rural households and communities, in particular those due to the effects of HIV/AIDS, and existing coping strategies; to identify how LSTs could assist in overcoming those; and to identify key factors necessary to improve the adoption of such technologies by poor rural women. The study was conducted in four communities from two districts in high HIV/AIDS prevalence areas in western Kenya. The report firstly presents an overview of the two districts in question, an introduction to the field sites and survey methods (most findings are based on Rapid Appraisal methods for data collection). Secondly, the main labour constraints facing the researched communities, their causes and effects are outlined, followed by a discussion of how those are exacerbated by HIV/AIDS once the epidemic's impact is felt by households and communities. Thirdly, initiatives already in place to help communities overcome their power constraints are outlined, followed by an identification of further opportunities for reducing the burden of labour constraints and farm power shortages on the most vulnerable households. Even if one does not share the reports overall belief in a technology-based solution to overcome HIV/AIDS induced problems of rural farming households, the report is a good starting point to consider the potential role of LSTs to mitigate HIV/AIDS impact or, even better, to help still 'intact' households to adopt such technologies before any impact is felt - which in both research districts, with HIV/AIDS prevalence rates well above the national average for Kenya, is bound to happen for the majority of households in the foreseeable future. The report's main conclusion is that it should be possible to alleviate the most pressing problems facing the farming community arising from labour constraints through the identification, dissemination and support of appropriate labour saving technologies and practices. In addition, with the growing changes in household composition - often triggered or at least exacerbated by HIV/AIDS - special attention has to be paid to addressing the particular needs of vulnerable groups.

Bishop-Sambrook, C., J. **Kienzle**, W. **Mariki**, M. **Owenya** and F. **Ribeiro** (2004) *Conservation Agriculture as a Labour Saving Practice for Vulnerable Households. A Study of the Suitability of Reduced Tillage and Cover Crops for Households under Labour Stress in Babati and Karatu Districts, Northern Tanzania*. Rome: International Fund for Agricultural Development (IFAD) and the United Nations Food and Agricultural Organisation (FAO).

This study has as its objective to determine the extent to which conservation farming practices are labour saving, and their suitability for use by vulnerable households. Two principal components within conservation agriculture are examined, reduced tillage and cover crops (RTCC). The findings are based on two types of data: on-farm field trials to generate labour and other input data associated with RTCC in comparison to conventional cultivation systems; and a qualitative review of farmers' reactions to conservation tillage equipment and practices in two districts in northern Tanzania. The findings - which should be taken as indicative of potential trends only as they are based on a comparatively small sample and one agricultural season only - include the following: While similar to experiences from settings in Latin America, land degradation has played a crucial role in sparking an interest in (some of the elements of) conservation agriculture, it may take the impact of HIV/AIDS combined with severe labour shortages to act as a catalyst for propelling African smallholders down the path towards conservation agriculture; results from the two sites suggest that it is possible to make significant savings in labour inputs when using RTCC technologies and practices - who benefits from such labour savings is household and often also gender specific; looking at cost, the RTCC cultivation system reduces the labour component of cost by substituting non-labour farm power inputs for labour - non-labour systems tend, however, to be more expensive, which has particular implications for the affordability of RTCC for poorer households (who at the same time might lose the opportunity to work as casual labourers on other people's farms); looking at reactions of vulnerable households to the introduction of RTCC, it was however found that poor female-headed households were among the most enthusiastic participants, as they were keen to overcome their labour constraints while at the same time the conduct of the study presented for many of them (who had little contact with extension services before) a unique opportunity to interact with researchers and extension staff which resulted in increased self-confidence among those farmers and greater respect towards them in the community.

Bonnard, P. (2002) *HIV/AIDS Mitigation: Using what we already know*. FANTA Technical Note No. **5**. Washington DC: Academy for Educational Development.

This short note sums up the main impacts of HIV/AIDS on food security and livelihood strategies and then discusses possible interventions derived more generally from food security and development programming. The main point made concerning the latter is that different strategies and interventions are bound to be relevant to different scenarios of how the pandemic is affecting a community. To design appropriate mitigation strategies it is thus important where a community is within the progression of the pandemic. A community with low HIV infection rates but a high concentration of risk factors might require a strategy emphasising prevention, such as the introduction of HIV/AIDS messages into agricultural extension programmes. In contrast, a community with high infection, morbidity and mortality rates might better benefits from new skills training for afflicted households. While very brief, this note is a good starting point to think in more detail about the issues involved in HIV/AIDS mitigation.

Bryceson, D., J. **Fonseca** and J. **Kadzandira** (2004) *Social Pathways from the HIV/AIDS Deadlock of Disease, Denial and Desperation in Rural Malawi*. Lilongwe: CARE Malawi.

This study explores recent social changes within rural households and communities in Lilongwe rural district in Malawi in the context of

HIV/AIDS. Community responses are traced corresponding to the three main stages of the HIV/AIDS cycle: infection and transmission; morbidity and death; and the aftermath of death, encompassing for example widowhood, orphanhood and household reconstitution. The ultimate objective of the study was to 'identify points of opportunity for the nurturing of social pathways that provide some hope for the future'. While the report is highly descriptive and one would have wished for a more to-the-point analysis, it does present valuable field data on matrilineal and patrilineal households and communities and raises a number of crucial issues that ask for more in-depth study. The latter include (among others that have often already been extensively discussed in the literature elsewhere, like the inferior social and economic position of women in comparison to men): a discussion of prevailing fatalism as disempowering and preventing people to become actors in their own right in combating HIV transmission; and a discussion of the unprecedented challenges rural Youth face in Malawi today which make them highly susceptible and vulnerable to HIV/AIDS. Taken together, the most valuable aspect of this report is its focus on social agency, based on the underlying assumption that individual health depends on broader social and community characteristics. The report ends with suggestions on how positive agency on the parts of different segments of the rural population in Malawi could be exercised within the three stages of the epidemic outlined above.

Chopra, M. (2003) *Equity Issues in HIV/AIDS, Nutrition and Food Security in Southern Africa*. Regional Network for Equity in Health in Southern Africa (EQUINET).

The paper starts from the observation that common health and agricultural services have not significantly reduced the vulnerability or susceptibility of rural people to HIV/AIDS, nor to food insecurity or malnutrition. HIV/AIDS, nutrition and food security are described as interacting at biological, individual, community and national levels, all four of which are linked and reinforce each other. It is suggested that greater awareness of the synergies between nutrition, food security and HIV/AIDS could lead to an approach in which prevention, treatment, rehabilitation and mitigation strategies are combined in ways that reduce vulnerability and susceptibility. The ultimate objective of such an approach must be enhanced resilience of livelihood systems to the epidemic.

---

du Guerny, J. (2002b) *Meeting the HIV/AIDS Challenge to Food Security. The role of labour saving technologies in farm-households.* Bangkok: United Nations Development Programme (UNDP) and United Nations Food and Agricultural Organisation (FAO).

This paper approaches the issue of labour saving technologies to mitigate HIV/AIDS impact from the perspective of food security at the farm-household level. It is based on the assumption that in HIV/AIDS afflicted or affected farm households, the nature of the household changes as AIDS induced morbidity and mortality takes its course. With every such change the farm household becomes less food secure and more vulnerable, as well as less of a production unit. As farm households move downwards on this scale of increasing vulnerability, mitigation strategies become ever more important - leading to the conundrum that households have less and less means to adopt LSTs at a time when they would need such LSTs most. For low prevalence countries the paper thus advocates the introduction of LSTs to farm households before HIV/AIDS possibly strikes, in order to make such households less susceptible and more resilient. More generally it is argued that in order to be effective, LST interventions in AIDS affected communities need to be tailored to take into account the changing nature of households over time - visible often in an increasing number of grandparent-, widow-, or widower-headed households. Equally, to be sustainable LST mitigation efforts need to be able to draw on long-term outside support both, from the community and from higher public levels. The paper further argues that the magnitude of the challenge HIV/AIDS poses depends on the type of farming system as well as a farm household's own resilience. The introduction of LSTs thus requires a two-track strategy by type of farming system as well as type of household. In addition, in view of the fact that the gender division of labour is intimately linked to the functioning of both, special attention to gender issues is advocated when introducing LSTs.

Food and Agriculture Organisation of the UN (FAO) (2003) *Mitigating the impact of HIV/AIDS on food security and rural poverty*. Rome: FAO HIV/AIDS Programme.

This report summarizes the contributions and discussions from a three-day meeting organised by the FAO and held in Rome in December 2001 with the objective to: develop a common understanding of HIV/AIDS impact on rural livelihoods; identify approaches to mitigate this impact; seek ways of integrating HIV-related activities into agricultural activities; and identify interventions to reduce the vulnerability of certain groups, including the very poor, widows and AIDS orphans. The report starts by summarising what is 'known' about the impact of HIV/AIDS on agriculture and food security and advocating a livelihoods framework to fully comprehend that impact. It then - and that is its most interesting part - gives examples of country experiences concerning strategies adopted and activities implemented to mitigate HIV/AIDS impact through the agricultural sector (case studies are represented from Cambodia, Lesotho, Tanzania, Uganda, Zimbabwe and Zambia). Overall, eight potential areas for agriculture-based responses were identified during the meeting and are discussed under the following headings, often exemplified by intervention examples from the above mentioned countries: labour saving technologies; knowledge preservation and transmission; rural institution and capacity building; gender equality; improving nutrition; social and economic safety nets; monitoring and evaluation of response strategies; and mainstreaming HIV/AIDS. The report ends with the usual call to move towards more effective partnerships between local, national and international stakeholders.

Hemrich, G. and B. **Schneider** (1997) *HIV/AIDS as a cross-sectoral issue for Technical Cooperation. Focus on agriculture and rural development*. Eschborn: Deutsche Gesellschaft für Technische Zusammenarbeit (GTZ).

This paper argues that as a cross-sectoral problem, HIV/AIDS is intrinsically linked to core technical areas of development work. In particular in high prevalence areas, technical cooperation projects of all kinds - even though the focus here is on agriculture and rural development - are potentially affected by the pandemic. Defining the linkage between HIV/AIDS and such projects as bi-directional, the report discusses how HIV/AIDS can affect non-health project work as well as how such project work might influence the course of the HIV/AIDS epidemic in a particular setting. The relevance of HIV/AIDS to non-health projects is hereby broken down into four categories: personal safety and professional competence of project staff; vulnerability of the target group to HIV infection and AIDS impact; linkages between HIV/AIDS and project objectives, strategies and activities; and HIV/AIDS-related management and personnel issues. The discussion is largely based on two case studies: an integrated food security programme in Eastern Province in Kenya, and a fisheries project in Malawi. While concentrating on project activities carried out by the Deutsche Gesellschaft für Technische Zusammenarbeit (GZT), the findings and recommendations are of potential relevance to a wider range of development cooperation activities.

Holden, S. (2003) *AIDS on the Agenda: Adapting Development and Humanitarian Programmes to Meet the Challenge of HIV.* Oxford: Oxfam.

This book is aimed at managers within the development business as well as policy makers and makes the case for mainstreaming AIDS into development and humanitarian programmes. In the first part of the publication, AIDS is discussed as a development issue, an issue that is not bound to disappear any time soon but will remain an entrenched problem for a long time to come, forcing development agencies to confront the challenges of containing and coping with HIV infection and the impacts of AIDS within their broader agendas. Such HIV/AIDS-aware responses are discussed at different levels, namely in terms of 'AIDS work', 'Integrated AIDS work', 'Mainstreaming AIDS internally', 'Mainstreaming AIDS externally' and as 'Complementary Partnerships'. These different approaches are defined in concrete and a number of examples given for each, including in the area of agricultural extension services. Some of those examples are based on hypothetical scenarios, others on case studies mainly drawn from three development agencies and their programmes in Africa: Action Aid, Oxfam GB, and Save the Children UK. While overall the book promotes the strategy of responding to AIDS indirectly, by making core humanitarian and development work relevant to the changes wrought by AIDS without necessarily doing 'AIDS work', to date 'AIDS work' dominates the global response and most concrete case scenarios thus fall into that category. In making the case for mainstreaming AIDS into development and humanitarian work, the book discusses how such work can have the adverse effect and increase susceptibility and vulnerability to HIV/AIDS instead of reducing it, as well as how the epidemic can undermine development and humanitarian work. The second part of the book then introduces experiences of mainstreaming AIDS internally and externally based on case studies from the three organisations mentioned above, while part three presents some general ideas for mainstreaming AIDS, again covering internal mainstreaming as well as external mainstreaming in development and humanitarian work.

Jayne, T., M. **Villarreal**, P. **Pingali** and G. **Hemrich** (2004) *Interactions between the Agricultural Sector and the HIV/AIDS Pandemic: Implications for Agricultural Policy*. Rome: United Nations Food and Agricultural Organisation (FAO).

This paper underscores the potentially central role of agricultural policy in mitigating the spread and impacts of the HIV/AIDS epidemic in the hardest-hit countries in eastern and southern Africa, and discusses how the design of such policies and programmes needs to be modified in the face of the epidemic. An introduction outlines the basic assumptions on which the paper is based, the most important of which is that agricultural growth is the catalyst for wider structural transformation and development, in particular in an African context where a majority of people earn the bulk of their income from agriculture-related activities (an assumption in itself questionable, see for example Ellis & Harris, 2004). The paper continues in discussing the current understanding of the effects of HIV/AIDS on agriculture and rural livelihoods, arguing for example that the evidence as to how AIDS is affecting agricultural systems and cropping patterns is mixed, and that loss of family labour due to premature death at household level does not necessarily imply that labour becomes the limiting input in agricultural production - from which follows that to focus on labour-saving agricultural technologies is not necessarily the appropriate policy response for agricultural research and extension systems. More broadly, it is argued that one of the most powerful tools at the disposal of agricultural policy makers is to put in place policies and programmes that generate broad based income growth and poverty reduction, as such policies bolster rural communities' resilience when the long-wave impacts of HIV/AIDS hit. The last section considers implications of this approach, centred on the belief that central to poverty alleviation are policies to promote agricultural growth. Illustrative examples of policies related to agriculture and rural development that may mitigate the impact of AIDS or reduce HIV transmission are then provided. These are grouped into four categories: policies affecting factor use and input markets; agricultural research and extension systems; commodity markets; and gender-differentiated resource allocation. The paper acknowledges that this is a rather broad list of proposals that would need refinement in the light of each country-specific context. It also appears to be the case that those four areas are given equal importance, whereas in reality certain types of policies - for example those relating to a change in gender-based resource allocation - need to predate or supplement other policy measures to make those successful.

Kim, J., J. **Gear**, J. **Hargreaves**, B. **Makhubele**, K. **Mashaba**, L. **Morison**, M. **Motsei**, C. **Peters**, J. **Porter**, P. **Pronyk** and C. **Watts** (2002) *Social Interventions for HIV/AIDS. Intervention with Microfinance for AIDS and Gender Equity*. Acornhoek, South Africa: Rural AIDS and Development Action Research Program.

This report discusses a multi-sectoral approach to HIV control, the Intervention with Microfinance for AIDS and Gender Equity (IMAGE) carried out in Sekhukhuneland, a densely settled rural area in Limpopo Province in South Africa. The overall aim of IMAGE is to develop an innovative approach to the prevention of HIV/AIDS that explicitly addresses the key structural factors driving the epidemic, such as poverty, gender-based violence, and broader gender inequalities. It is thus based on an ecological framework in order to understand the interplay of personal, situational and socio-cultural factors that combine to create patterns of vulnerability, shifting the focus of intervention from concepts of individual risk to those of creating an enabling environment. In concrete, the IMAGE intervention integrates and mainstreams a programme of gender and HIV education into an existing microfinance initiative in order to create an enabling environment for behavioural change. The intervention as described here in detail thus comprises two distinct but inter-related parts: a microfinance programme, and gender and HIV training. The report outlines how such group-based, integrated interventions might not only empower women economically but enhance their well-being, their social status and autonomy, and thus transform the vulnerability context for HIV transmission and impact mitigation.

Kraak, V., D. **Pelletier**, E. **Frongillo** and S. **Rajabiun** (1999) *The Potential Role of Food Aid for AIDS Mitigation in East Africa. Stakeholder Views*. Washington DC: Academy for Educational Development.

This report explores the circumstances and conditions under which external food aid might enhance the mitigation efforts of households and communities in response to HIV/AIDS in Kenya and Uganda. It is based on a series of interviews with local and international organisations, government officials and other stakeholders in both countries who are active in food aid and/or HIV/AIDS prevention and mitigation. The main conclusion is that food aid may play a key role in the AIDS mitigation process in some circumstances in which the situations in which it is to be used are clearly defined. Such clarification needs to involve establishing criteria or indicators for targeting food aid, determining the most effective delivery mechanisms, defining appropriate time frames, and determining when external aid or local purchases are most advantageous. More generally, food aid is more likely to contribute to sustained mitigation if it is part of a larger development effort (not predominately regarded as a humanitarian assistance measure).

Lundberg, M., M. **Over** and P. **Mujinja** (2000) 'Sources of Financial Assistance for Households Suffering an Adult Death in Kagera, Tanzania', *The South African Journal of Economics* **68**, pp. 947-984.

This paper, based on a panel dataset from Kagera region in Tanzania, examines household responses to death with a special focus on

HIV/AIDS. It does so in looking at households' receipts of transfers and other unearned income around a death. Three sources of financial assistance available to households following a death are identified: private transfers; private borrowing; and assistance from public or other formal organisations. Findings include that resource abundant households receive more private transfers, whereas resource-poor households rely relatively more on credit. Resource-abundant households are thus wealthy not only in terms of physical and human assets, but also in social capital, as they have larger networks on whom they can depend in times of crisis. Poor households find it hard to receive private assistance, making the impact of death potentially worse as they are not only hit harder, but must bear a larger part of the burden alone. These findings raise policy questions, such as whether micro-credit programmes may be a useful tool in helping resource-poor households to cope with the impact of adult death in areas hard-hit by the AIDS epidemic.

Meinert, L., M. **Whyte**, S. **Reynolds-Whyte** and B. **Kyaddondo** (2003) 'Faces of Globalisation. AIDS and ARV Medicine in Uganda', *FOLK* **45**, pp. 105-123.

In this article a distinction is made between globalisation as background, defined by the analyst, and globalisation as context, defined by the actor involved. Three cases of people living with AIDS in Uganda, all three with access to ART, are discussed. Globalisation has different consequences and meanings within each of their contexts. In the first case, the global aspect of anti-retroviral medicine is not relevant for the actor, but she interprets her illness and her access to medication in the context of strained family relations, insufficient food production, and moral obligations. In the second case, different forms of globalisation form part of the actor's context and are actively influenced and shaped by him and vice versa. In the third case, the actors were part of someone else's global project, but took the opportunity this access offered and let it work to their advantage. The article is a very good example of how enquiring about people's own sense of connections and priorities allows to see how differently local actors draw global connections and inspirations into their lived realities.

Mutangadura, G., D. **Mukurazita** and H. **Jackson** (1999) *A Review of household and community responses to the HIV/AIDS epidemic in the rural areas of sub-Saharan Africa.* UNAIDS Best Practice Collection. Geneva: UNAIDS.

This study is a desk review and analysis of relevant literature on household and community coping responses to HIV/AIDS at the time of writing with the objective to make policy recommendations. Three types of strategies behind afflicted or affected households' responses are identified: strategies aimed at improving food security; strategies aimed at raising income in order to maintain expenditure patterns; and strategies aimed at alleviating labour loss. Concerning community responses, the study shows (with the help of case study examples from different settings in sub-Saharan Africa) how community initiatives have successfully sprung up to mitigate the impact of HIV/AIDS. Those responses either take the form of traditional grassroots organisations, or more formal community-based organisations relying on external support. The responses by traditional grassroots organisations documented here have their strength not only in being cost-effective, but equally and arguably more crucially in being based on local needs and available resources as well as on the mutual understanding of community members - which is not always the case concerning responses dependent on external support. Their main limitation is that they cannot generate enough resources to for example make drugs and other care available to ill members, and may place a heavy burden on women's working time. In high prevalence areas such grassroots organisations might also become increasingly under strain. More generally it is argued that relief support to afflicted and affected households must be combined with and eventually replaced with mitigation support for the longer term. This requires investment in human development to eventually achieve the basic well-being of national populations - the latter task calling for meaningful partnerships between communities, governments, donors, international and national NGOs and the private sector.

O'Donnell, M. (2004) *Food Security, Livelihoods and HIV/AIDS. A Guide to the Linkages, Measurements and Programming Implications*. London: Save the Children UK.

This report is meant as a guide mainly for development practitioners, but its three different sections can be useful to anybody involved in HIV/AIDS research or mitigation activities. The first section discusses HIV/AIDS and food security linkages and provides an overview for those not familiar with the literature in this area. The second section on methodology is particularly useful and intended for those who consider carrying out research into those linkages, as well as for programme managers for whom guidance on evaluating the quality of such research is important. The final section deals with linking research to interventions in order to decide on best-practice mitigation strategies.

Page, S. (1999) 'The Need for a Paradigm Shift towards Farmer Participatory Research and Training in the Interest of Zimbabwe's AIDS Survivors'. Paper presented at the Conference AIDS, Livelihood and Social Change in Africa, 15-16 April 1999, Wageningen University and Research Centre.

This paper - looking at the case of Zimbabwe - argues that the conventional approach to agricultural research and extension services is becoming irrelevant as a result of the AIDS pandemic. The development of appropriate survival strategies for in particular female smallholders will in fact require a substantial paradigm shift on the part of research and extension. The main objectives within such a new paradigm should be the promotion of food security at household level, the reduction of poverty throughout the community, and the rehabilitation of the environment. The new paradigm should thus be concerned with low input agriculture and involve farmers in both, the planning and implementation process. Farmer Field Schools are advocated as the most suitable form for farmer participatory research, as they provide an opportunity to build on indigenous knowledge in the process of developing sustainable agricultural practices.

Richey, L. and S. **Haakonsson** (2004) *Access to ARV Treatment: Aid, Trade and Governance in Uganda*. Danish Institute for International Studies (DIIS) Working Paper **2004/19**. Copenhagen: DIIS.

This paper argues that access to ARVs for AIDS treatment creates a field binding local and global governance. Using the example of Uganda it is shown how local modalities of AIDS treatment are governed by the context of global trade through the implementation of patents on medicine in the WTO, as well as by the context of global aid through development assistance. The same countries that provide aid to fight AIDS in developing countries use the WTO to prevent those countries from accessing cheap (generic) medicines. The paper examines the Ugandan case in terms of how the disconnect between international and national priorities on the one hand, and between aid and trade on the other is affecting access to ARVs. It argues that despite the many interventions addressing HIV/AIDS and dramatic price reductions in the price of ARVs even in the in many ways 'best practice' example of Uganda only a minority of the infected population in need is receiving treatment, and promises of wider treatment coverage for all who need it are unrealistic within the prevailing global system.

Shadlen, K. (2004) 'Challenges to Treatment: The Price-Infrastructure Trap and Access to HIV/AIDS Drugs', *Journal of International Development* **16**, pp. 1169-1180.

This paper discusses issues in international political economy that affect responses to the HIV/AIDS pandemic in the developing world. Its main argument is that stable access to affordable medication is essential for developing countries' mitigation responses in an overall environment in which treatment is becoming increasingly regarded as essential to any such response. It is argued that developing countries must overcome what is called the 'price-infrastructure trap', where high drug prices reduce the feasibility of scaling-up treatment programmes, such reduced feasibility creates disincentives to invest in public health infrastructure, and poor health infrastructure limits the effectiveness of even small-scale treatment programmes. Four mechanisms for increasing development countries' access to affordable medication are discussed and the political economy obstacles inherent in each of those examined, with particular emphasis on the impediments posed by the global regime on intellectual property rights.

Topouzis, D. and J. **du Guerny** (1999) *Sustainable Agricultural/Rural Development and Vulnerability to the AIDS Epidemic.* Rome: United Nations Food and Agricultural Organisation (FAO) and United Nations Development Programme (UNDP).

This report discusses the rural dimension of susceptibility and vulnerability to HIV/AIDS and how agricultural and rural development projects might contribute to reducing it. It is based on seven case studies of agricultural/rural development projects and programmes operating in countries with high, medium and low HIV prevalence respectively (study sites are: Cambodia, Ghana, a joint project in Chad and Cameroon, Tanzania, Zambia, Zimbabwe, and a joint project in Zimbabwe, Malawi, Zambia and Mozambique). While many of the case studies illustrate the complexity of establishing cause and effect relationships between HIV and rural development projects, such projects are shown to - often indirectly - influence the vulnerability context of the livelihood systems of rural households and with it susceptibility and vulnerability to HIV/AIDS positively or negatively. The relevance of rural development projects as catalysts for reducing susceptibility and vulnerability to HIV/AIDS is discussed in relation to poverty, food insecurity, gender inequality and migration. The report ends by outlining possible strategies to integrate an HIV/AIDS component into rural development projects with the overall objective of transforming the wider susceptibility and vulnerability context.

United States Agency for International Development (USAID) (2003) *Multisectoral Responses to HIV/AIDS. A Compendium of Promising Practices from Africa.* Washington DC: Academy for Educational Development.

This publication introduces a collection of 22 promising practices in response to the HIV/AIDS pandemic from 13 private voluntary organisations (PVOs) working in sub-Saharan Africa. These practices are presented under the following headings: Agriculture, food security and nutrition; capacity and human resources development; care and support; children; conflict and humanitarian relief; democracy and governance; economic development and microfinance; and education. Most of the practices discussed here are very young, they thus do not have measurable results yet and cannot be termed 'best practices'. But it is hoped that their documentation will enhance general knowledge on how to respond to HIV/AIDS as a major development issue.

White, J. and J. **Morton** (2005) 'Mitigating impacts of HIV/AIDS on rural livelihoods: NGO experiences in sub-Saharan Africa', *Development in Practice* **15**, pp. 186-199.

This paper argues that HIV/AIDS has exposed the inadequacies of standard development strategies, in particular their failure to secure the livelihood needs of vulnerable rural population groups. At the same time it is observed that many local initiatives have begun to tackle the effects of the HIV/AIDS pandemic on rural communities. The paper then looks in more detail at nine NGO projects in four countries - Uganda, Tanzania, Zimbabwe and Lesotho (see also White, 2002). Those projects are in the fields of agriculture, skill training and microfinance, often combined with offering home care and support. Factors of success identified include the use of participatory processes to identify target groups, and the involvement of local political leaders and adults trusted by young people in project activities. Main challenges are seen in improving monitoring systems, effectively disseminating lessons learned to wider stakeholders, and persuading donors to support holistic livelihood interventions as a matter of urgency. The paper further urges caution in the process of 'scaling up' interventions that have been successful in one particular setting, as experience has revealed the importance of responding to the concrete needs identified by local communities as well as of adapting successful approaches to the particular circumstances in which new interventions are to take place.

White, J. (ed.) (2002) *Facing the Challenge. NGO experiences of mitigating the impacts of HIV/AIDS in sub-Saharan Africa*. Greenwich: Natural Resource Institute.

This report starts from the observation that AIDS-affected communities and NGOs have been at the forefront of responding to the impacts of the HIV/AIDS pandemic and many innovative local projects have emerged. Those have, however, rarely been written up and publicized among a wider audience. To counter this shortcoming, nine case studies collected from Uganda, Tanzania, Zimbabwe and Lesotho are presented here in detail, usually written up by local project staff and then edited by the author. One objective of this report was initially to identify possible 'best practice' approaches in relation to responding to the impact of HIV/AIDS. It was, however, found that this will only be possible once more systematic monitoring and evaluation systems are put in place. The value of this overview is thus in documenting and analysing the projects presented here which can all be called successful. More generally, the report confirms that local organisations and NGOs, be they community based or parts of a wider network, are spearheading the response to the epidemic (see also Barnett & Grellier, 2003). In many of the cases presented here, such responses were not specifically related to HIV/AIDS only but reflected wider problems of poverty and vulnerability, revealing how critical it is to tackle existing poverty and resource constraints while at the same time understanding the interplay between HIV/AIDS and prevailing problems. Often, project activities were equally relevant to all members of a beneficiary community who are experiencing poverty, raising critical questions about targeting development activities in HIV/AIDS communities at PLWHA. Overall it is concluded that any development initiative in a region with significant HIV prevalence will, whether knowingly or not, interact with the impact of the pandemic. A lack of understanding of the complex dynamics between HIV/AIDS and poverty may thus exacerbate problems of poverty and underdevelopment further.

Additional sources

Adjé-Touré, C., R. Cheingsong, J. Garcìa-Lerma, S. Eholié, M.-Y. Borget, J.-M. Bouchez, R. Otten, C. Maurice, M. Sassan-Morokro, R. Ekpini, M. Nolan, T. Chorba, W. Heneine and J. Nkengasong (2003) 'Antiretroviral therapy in HIV-2-infected patients: changes in plasma viral load, CD4+ cell counts, and drug resistance profiles of patients treated in Abidjan, Côte d'Ivoire', *AIDS* **17**, pp. S49-S54.

Armstrong, S. (2003) *Stepping back from the edge. The pursuit of antiretroviral therapy in Botswana, South Africa and Uganda*. UNAIDS Best Practice Collection. Geneva: UNAIDS.

Barnett, T., T. Fantan, B. Mbakile and A. Whiteside (2002) *The private sector responds to the epidemic: Debswana-a global benchmark*. UNAIDS Best Practice Collection. Geneva: UNAIDS.

Beeker, C., C. Guenther-Grey and A. Raj (1998) 'Community Empowerment Paradigm Drift and the Primary Prevention of HIV/AIDS', Social Science and Medicine **46**, pp. 831-842.

Bellos, A. (2001) 'Roche bows to Brazil on AIDS drug' *The Guardian*, 1 September 2001.

Berwick, D. (2002) '"We all have AIDS": case for reducing the cost of HIV drugs to zero', *British Medical Journal* **324**, pp. 214-216.

Bishop-Sambrook, C. (2003a) 'HIV/AIDS Susceptibility and Vulnerability Pathway: A Tool for Identifying Indicators, Role Models and Innovations'. Paper presented at the Technical Consultation on Measuring Vulnerability in the Light of the HIV/AIDS Pandemic at the UN Regional Inter-Agency Coordination and Support Office, 9-11 September 2003, Johannesburg.

Block, R. (2001) 'Daimler Provides AIDS Help to Employees in South Africa', *Wall Street Journal*, 19 June 2001.

Blower, S. and P. Farmer (2003) 'Predicting the public health impact of antiretrovirals: preventing HIV in developing countries', *AIDScience* **3** (11). http://www.aidscience.org/Articles/aidscience033.asp, accessed 18 April 2005.

Bredewold, M. (2004) *Mozambique. Report on Visit to Pilot Project on Junior Farmer Field and Life Schools*. Pietermaritzburg, South Africa: Farmer Support Group.

British Broadcasting Corporation (BBC) (22 March 2005) 'India backs cheap drug clampdown.'

British Broadcasting Corporation (BBC) (18 March 2005) 'India facing new drugs patent law.'

British Broadcasting Corporation (BBC) (19 November 2003) 'The Brazilian Model - Recife.'

British Broadcasting Corporation (BBC) (18 November 2003) 'Food aid to target HIV sufferers.'

British Broadcasting Corporation (BBC) (6 September 2003) 'Brazil issues AIDS drug threat.'

British Broadcasting Corporation (BBC) (14 July 2003) 'Brazil's pioneering AIDS programme.'

British Broadcasting Corporation (BBC) (23 August 2001) 'Brazil to break AIDS patent.'

Campbell, C. (2003) *'Letting Them Die'. Why HIV/AIDS Prevention Programmes Fail.* Oxford: James Currey.

Christian Aid (2004) *If not now, when? HIV, drugs and prevention*. London: Christian Aid.

Coriat, B., J. Dumoulin, Y.-A. Flori, T. Barnett, Y. Souteyrand and J.-P. Moatti (2003) 'Patents, Generic Drugs and the Market for Antiretrovirals', in Agence Nationale de Recherches sur le SIDA (ANRS) (ed.) *Economics of AIDS and Access to HIV/AIDS Care in Developing Countries. Issues and Challenges*, pp. 27-37. Paris: ANRS.

Desclaux, A., I. Lanièce, I. Ndoye and B. Taverne (2002) *L'initiative sénégalaise d'accès aux médicaments antirétroviraux. Analyses économiques, sociales, comportementales et médicales*. Paris: Agence Nationale de Recherches sur le SIDA (ANRS).

Djomand, G., T. Roels, T. Ellerbrock, D. Hanson, F. Diomande, B. Monga, C. Maurice, J. Nkengasong, R. Konan-Koko, A. Kadio, S. Wiktor, E. Lackritz, J. Saba and T. Chorba (2003) 'Virologic and immunologic outcomes and programmatic challenges of an antiretroviral treatment pilot project in Abidjan, Côte d'Ivoire', *AIDS* **17**, pp. S5-S15.

Donahue, J. (1998) *Community-Based Economic Support for Households Affected by HIV/AIDS*. Arlington, VA: US Agency for International Development (USAID).

du Guerny, J. (2002a) *Agriculture and HIV/AIDS*. New York: United Nations Development Programme (UNDP).

du Guerny, J., L.-N. Hsu and S. Chitna (2002) *Farmer Life Schools. A Development Strategy to Empower Rural Farmers and Prevent HIV*. Bangkok: United Nations Development Programme (UNDP) and United Nations Food and Agricultural Organisation (FAO).

Durier, N. (2003) 'Treatment of HIV Disease with Highly Active Antiretroviral Therapy (HAART) in Chiradzulu District, Malawi', *Antiviral Therapy* **8**, S211(Abstract).

Egal, F. and A. Valstar (1999) 'HIV/AIDS and nutrition: Helping families and communities to cope', *Food, Nutrition and Agriculture* **25**, pp. 20-26.

Eholie, S.-P., M. Nolan, A. Gaumon, J. Mambo, Y. Kouamé-Yebouet, R. Aka-Kakou, E. Bissagnene and A. Kadio (2003) 'Antiretroviral Treatment can be Cost-saving for Industry and Life-saving for Workers: a Case Study from Côte d'Ivoire's Private Sector', in Agence Nationale de Recherches sur le SIDA (ANRS) (ed.) *Economics of AIDS and Access to HIV/AIDS Care in Developing Countries. Issues and Challenges*, pp. 329-346. Paris: ANRS.

Farmer, P., F. Léandre, J. Mukherjee, M. Claude, P. Nevil, M. Smith-Fawzi, S. Koenig, A. Castro, M. Becerra, J. Sachs, A. Attaran and J. Kim (2001) 'Community-based approaches to HIV treatment in resource-poor settings', *The Lancet* **358**, pp. 404-409.

Feuer, C. (2004) 'HIV Drugs Trickle Into Uganda', *AMFAR Treatment Insider* **5**, p. 6.

Freedberg, K. and Y. Yazdanpanah (2003) 'Cost-effectiveness of HIV Therapies in Resource-Poor Countries', in Agence Nationale de Recherches sur le SIDA (ANRS) (ed.) *Economics of AIDS and Access to HIV/AIDS Care in Developing Countries. Issues and Challenges*, pp. 267-291. Paris: ANRS.

Galvão, J. (2002) 'Access to antiretroviral drugs in Brazil', *The Lancet* **360**, pp. 1862-1865.

Gari, J. (2002) *Agrobiodiversity, food security and HIV/AIDS mitigation in sub-Saharan Africa.* Rome: United Nations Food and Agricultural Organisation (FAO).

Gray, R., X. Li, M. Wawer, S. Gange, D. Serwadda, N. Sewankambo, R. Moore, F. Wabwire-Mangen, T. Lutalo and T. Quinn (2003) 'Stochastic simulation of the impact of antiretroviral therapy and HIV vaccines on HIV transmission; Rakai, Uganda', *AIDS* **17**, pp. 1941-1951.

Gruber, J. and M. Caffrey (2005) 'HIV/AIDS and community conflict in Nigeria: implications and challenges', *Social Science & Medicine* **60**, pp. 1209-1218.

Harvey, P. (2003) *HIV/AIDS: What are the implications for humanitarian action? A Literature Review*. London: Overseas Development Institute, Humanitarian Policy Group.

Heise, L. and C. Elias (1995) 'Transforming AIDS Prevention to Meet Women's Needs: A Focus on Developing Countries', *Social Science and Medicine* **40**, pp. 931-943.

Kadiyala, S. and S. Gillespie (2003) *Rethinking Food Aid to Fight AIDS*. Washington DC: International Food Policy Research Institute (IFPRI).

Katzenstein, D., M. Laga and J.-P. Moatti (2003) 'The evaluation of the HIV/AIDS Drug Access Initiatives in Côte d'Ivoire, Senegal and Uganda: how access to antiretroviral treatment can become feasible in Africa', *AIDS* **17**, pp. S1-S4.

Laurent, C., N. Diakhaté, N. Gueye, A. Touré, S. Sow, A. Faye, M. Gueye, I. Lanièce, C. Kane, F. Liégeois, L. Vergne, S. Mboup, S. Badiane, I. Ndoye and E. Delaporte (2002) 'The Senegalese government's highly active antiretroviral therapy initiative: an 18-month follow-up study', *AIDS* **16**, pp. 1363-1370.

Loevinsohn, M. and S. Gillespie (2003) *HIV/AIDS and the Food Crises in Southern Africa: An Agenda for Action Research and Learning How to Respond.* Washington DC: RENEWAL.

Lundberg, M. and M. Over (2000) 'Transfers and Household Welfare in Kagera', draft. http://www.iaen.org/conferences/durbansym/papers/38lundbergtext.pdf, accessed 18 April 2005.

MacNeil, J., F. Mberesero and G. Kilonzo (1999) 'Is care and support associated with preventive behaviour among people with HIV?', *AIDS CARE* **11**, pp. 537-546.

Marston, B. and K. de Cock (2004) 'Multivitamins, Nutrition, and Antiretroviral Therapy for HIV Disease in Africa', *The New England Journal of Medicine* **351**, pp. 78-80.

Moatti, J.-P., J. Prudhomme, D. Traore, A. Juillet-Amari, H. Akribi, P. Msellati and the Côte d'Ivoire Drug Access Initiative Socio-Behavioural Evaluation Group (2003a) 'Access to antiretroviral treatment and sexual behaviours of HIV-infected patients aware of their serostatus in Côte d'Ivoire', *AIDS* **17**, pp. S69-S77.

Moatti, J.-P., T. Barnett, Y. Souteyrand, Y.-A. Flori, J. Dumoulin and B. Coriat (2003b) 'Financing Efficient HIV Care and Antiretroviral Treatment to Mitigate the Impact of the AIDS Epidemic on Economic and Human Development', in Agence Nationale de Recherches sur le SIDA (ANRS) (ed.) *Economics of AIDS and Access to HIV/AIDS Care in Developing Countries. Issues and Challenges*, pp. 247-265. Paris: ANRS.

Mukherjee, J., P. Farmer, D. Niyizonkiza, L. McCorkle, C. Vanderwarker, P. Teixeira and J. Kim (2003) 'Tackling HIV in resource poor countries', *British Medical Journal* **327**, pp. 1104-1106.

Munthali, A. (2002) *Adaptive Strategies and Coping Mechanisms of Families and Communities Affected by HIV/AIDS in Malawi*. Geneva: United Nations Research Institute for Social Development (UNRISD).

Nyamukapa, C. and S. Gregson (2005) 'Extended family's and women's roles in safeguarding orphans' education in AIDS-afflicted rural Zimbabwe', *Social Science & Medicine* **60**, pp. 2155-2167.

Okoth, J., G. Khisa and J. Thomas (2002) 'Towards a holistic Farmer Field School approach for East Africa', *Leisa* **18**, pp. 18-19.

Orsi, F., L. Hasenclever, B. Fialho, P. Tigre and B. Coriat (2003) 'Intellectual Property Rights, Anti-AIDS Policy and Generic Drugs. Lessons from the Brazilian Public Health Programme', in Agence Nationale de Recherches sur le SIDA (ANRS) (ed.) *Economics of AIDS and Access to HIV/AIDS Care in Developing Countries. Issues and Challenges*, pp. 109-135. Paris: ANRS.

Page, S. (2001) 'Promoting the Survival of Rural Mothers with HIV/AIDS: A development strategy for southern Africa', *Development* **44**, pp. 40-46.

Page, S. and F. Nyakanda (2003) *How to Live Positively. A practical manual for facilitating community action in HIV/AIDS-affected areas*. Egham, Surrey: CABI Bioscience.

Panos Institute (2000) *Beyond Our Means? The cost of treating HIV/AIDS in the developing world*. London: Panos Institute.

Richards, P. (1999) 'Hurry, we are all dying of AIDS: Linking cultural and agro-technological responses to the challenge of living with HIV/AIDS in Africa'. Paper presented at the Conference AIDS, Livelihood and Social Change in Africa, 15-16 April 1999, Wageningen University and Research Centre.

Robins, S. and B. von Lieres (2004) 'AIDS Activism and Globalisation from Below: Occupying New Spaces of Citizenship in Post-apartheid South Africa', *IDS Bulletin* **35**, pp. 84-90.

Sauerborn, R., A. Adams and M. Hien (1996) 'Household Strategies to Cope with the Economic Cost of Illness', *Social Science and Medicine* **43**, pp. 291-301.

Smith, K. and S. Watkins (2005) 'Perceptions of risk and strategies for prevention: responses to HIV/AIDS in rural Malawi', *Social Science & Medicine* **60**, pp. 649-660.

Sokunthea, N. (2002) *The empowerment of Farmer Life Schools*. Phnom Penh: United Nations Development Programme (UNDP) and United Nations Food and Agricultural Organisation (FAO).

Steiner, K., J. Kienzle and F. Ribeiro (2004) *Mitigating the impact of HIV/AIDS by labour saving technologies*. African Conservation Tillage Network Information Series No. **9**. Harare: African Conservation Tillage Network (ACT).

Teixeira, P., M. Vitória and J. Barcarolo (2003) 'The Brazilian Experience in Providing Universal Access to Antiretroviral Therapy', in Agence Nationale de Recherches sur le SIDA (ANRS) (ed.) *Economics of AIDS and Access to HIV/AIDS Care in Developing Countries. Issues and Challenges*, pp. 69-88. Paris: ANRS.

Topouzis, D. (1998) *The Implications of HIV/AIDS for Rural Development Policy and Programming: Focus on Sub-Saharan Africa*. Rome: United Nations Food and Agricultural Organisation (FAO) and United Nations Development Programme (UNDP).

UNAIDS (2002) *HIV Voluntary Counselling and Testing: a gateway to prevention and care*. UNAIDS Best Practice Collection. Geneva: UNAIDS.

UNAIDS (1997) *Tuberculosis and AIDS*. UNAIDS Best Practice Collection. Geneva: UNAIDS.

United Nations Development Programme (UNDP) and Food and Agriculture Organisation of the UN (FAO) (2004) *Farmers' Life School Manual*. Bangkok: UNDP and FAO.

van der Ende, M., J. Prins, K. Brinkman, M. Keuter, J. Veenstra, S. Danner, H. Niesters, A. Osterhaus and M. Schutten (2003) 'Clinical, immunological and virological response to different antiretroviral regimens in a cohort of HIV-2-infected patients', *AIDS* **17**, pp. S55-S61.

Vermuelen, A. (2004) 'South Africa and the corporate fightback against AIDS', *Student Accountant*, published 5 March 2004. http://www.acca.org.uk/publications/studentaccountant/1107093, accessed 18 April 2005.

World Bank (2002) *Education and HIV/AIDS. A Window of Hope.* Washington DC: World Bank.

World Health Organisation (WHO) (2003) *Treating 3 Million By 2005. Making it happen.* Geneva: WHO.

Yech, P. (2003) 'Farmer Life Schools in Cambodia', *Leisa* **19**, pp. 11-12.

3. Other readings

On HIV/AIDS surveys:

Afrobarometer (April 2004) 'Public Opinion and HIV/AIDS: Facing Up to the Future?', retrieved from http://www.afrobarometer.org, accessed 24 February 2005.

Pettifor, A., H. Rees, A. Steffenson, L. Hlongwa-Madikizela, C. MacPhail, K. Vermaak and I. Kleinschmidt (2004) *HIV and Sexual Behaviour Among Young South Africans: A national survey of 15-24 year olds*. Johannesburg: Reproductive Health Research Unit, University of the Witwatersrand.

Shisana, O. and L. Simbayi (2002) *Nelson Mandela/HSRC Study of HIV/AIDS. South African National HIV Prevalence, Behavioural Risks and Mass Media. Household Survey 2002*. Cape Town: Human Sciences Research Council (HSRC) Publishers.

On urban-rural relations, poverty reduction and modernisation processes:

Bahiigwa, G., D. Rigby and P. Woodhouse (2004) 'Right Target, Wrong Mechanism? Agricultural Modernization and Poverty Reduction in Uganda', *World Development* **33**, pp. 481-496.

Blackden, M. and S. Canagarajah (2003) 'Gender and Growth in Africa: Evidence and Issues'. Paper presented at the World Bank UNECA Expert Meeting on Pro-Poor Growth, 23-24 June 2003, Kampala, Uganda.

Commission for Africa (2005) *Our Common Interest. Report of the Commission for Africa*. London: Commission for Africa.

This report is based on an initiative by British Prime Minister Tony Blair who in 2004 brought together 17 people - a majority from Africa where they have experiences as political leaders, public servants or in the private sector - to form a Commission for Africa, with the task to define the challenges facing the continent and to provide clear recommendations on how to initiate the changes needed to overcome poverty and deprivation on the continent. The concrete objective behind this report is to use the British presidency of the G8 and European Union during 2005 as a platform to push for the delivery and implementation of existing international commitments towards Africa, coupled with offering a fresh perspective on Africa and its diverse cultures and helping fulfil African aspirations for the future as formulated by African people themselves. The report has two parts: The first part, called 'the argument', is addressed to a wider audience and makes the case why urgent action on Africa is required and will ultimately benefit the whole global community. The second part, called 'analysis and evidence', lays out the sustenance and basis of the recommendations advocated by the commission, which are set out between those two sections. Whether one agrees with the analysis or the recommendations based on it or not, the second part provides a comprehensive source of information on all aspects of African development and suggestions on how to overcome development failures under the following headings: the case for action; lost decades: legacy and causes; through African eyes: culture; getting systems right: governance and capacity building; the need for peace and security; leaving no-one out: investing in people (this is the section where HIV/AIDS is discussed); going for growth and poverty reduction; more trade and fairer trade; where will the money come from: resources; and making it happen. Key recommendations centre on the strengthening of state capacity and the improvement of governance, and a doubling of international aid coupled with debt relief and other inventive schemes to provide the resources necessary to kick-start development in Africa.

Committee of Inquiry into a Comprehensive System of Social Security for South Africa (2002) *Transforming the Present - Protecting the Future*. Pretoria: Department of Social Development, Government of the Republic of South Africa.

de Ferranti, D., G. Perry, W. Foster, D. Lederman and A. Valdés (2005) *Beyond the City: The Rural Contribution to Development*. Washington DC: World Bank.

Devereux, S. (2002) 'Can Social Safety Nets Reduce Chronic Poverty?', *Development Policy Review* **20**, pp. 657-675.

Dorward, A. (2003) *Modelling Poor Farm-Household Livelihoods in Malawi: Lessons for Pro-Poor Policy*, draft. London: Imperial College London.

Ellis, F. (2000) *Rural Livelihoods and Diversity in Developing Countries*. Oxford: Oxford University Press.

Ellis, F. and N. Harris (2004) 'New Thinking About Urban and Rural Development'. Keynote Paper for the DFID Sustainable Development Retreat, 13 July 2004, University of Surrey, Guildford.

Food and Agriculture Organisation of the UN (FAO) (2004) *The State of Food Insecurity in the World 2004*. Rome: FAO.

Hanmer, L., G. Pyatt and H. White (1999) 'What do the World Bank's Poverty Assessments teach us about Poverty in sub-Saharan Africa?', *Development and Change* **30**, pp. 795-823.

James, D. (2001) 'Land for the Landless: Conflicting Images of Rural and Urban in South Africa's Land Reform Programme', *Journal of Contemporary African Studies* **19**, pp. 93-109.

Johnston, B. and P. Kilby (1975) *Agriculture and Structural Transformation. Economic Strategies in Late-Developing Countries.* New York: Oxford University Press.

Leavy, J. and H. White (2000) 'Rural Labour Markets and Poverty in sub-Saharan Africa'. Paper presented at the Development Studies Association Development Economics Study Group Conference, April 2000, Nottingham University.

Lipton, M. (1977) *Why Poor People Stay Poor. A study of urban bias in world development.* London: Temple Smith.

May, J. (2001) 'An Elusive Consensus: Definitions, measurement and analysis of poverty', in United Nations Development Programme (UNDP) (ed.) *Choices for the Poor: Lessons from National Poverty Strategies*, pp. 23-54. New York: UNDP.

Mellor, J. (1976) *The New Economics of Growth. A Strategy for India and the Developing World.* Ithaca, NY: Cornell University Press.

Quisumbing, A., L. Haddad, R. Meinzen-Dick and L. Brown (1998) 'Gender Issues for Food Security in Developing Countries: Implications for Project Design and Implementation', *Canadian Journal of Development Studies* **XIX** Special Issue, pp. 185-208.

Reardon, T. (1997) 'Using Evidence of Household Income Diversification to Inform Study of the Rural Nonfarm Labour Market in Africa', *World Development* **25**, pp. 735-747.

Sachs, J. (2005) *Investing in Development. A Practical Plan to Achieve the Millennium Development Goals.* London and Sterling, VA: Earthscan.

Scanlan, S. (2004) 'Women, Food Security, and Development in Less-Industrialized Societies: Contributions and Challenges for the New Century', *World Development* **32**, pp. 1807-1829.

United Nations General Assembly (18 September 2000) United Nations Millennium Declaration, A/RES/55/2.

World Bank (1996) *Taking Action for Poverty Reduction in sub-Saharan Africa. Report of an African Region Task Force.* Washington DC: World Bank.

On HIV/AIDS, governance and international relations:

Boone, C. and J. Batsell (2001) 'Politics and AIDS in Africa: Research Agendas in Political Science and International Relations', *Africa Today* **48**, pp. 3-33.

de Waal, A. (2003) 'How Will HIV/AIDS Transform African Governance?', *African Affairs* **102**, pp. 1-23.

Fukuyama, F. (2004) *State-Building. Governance and World Order in the 21st Century.* Ithaca, NY: Cornell University Press.

Manning, R. (2002) *AIDS and Democracy: What Do We Know? A Literature Review.* Durban, South Africa: Health Economics and HIV/AIDS Research Division (HEARD), University of Natal.

Moran, D. (2004) 'HIV/AIDS, Governance and Development: The Public Administration Factor', *Public Administration and Development* **24**, pp. 7-18.

On disease and social inequalities:

Farmer, P. (1996) 'Social Inequalities and Emerging Infectious Diseases', *Emerging Infectious Diseases* **2**, pp. 259-269.

Wilkinson, R. (1996) *Unhealthy Societies. The Afflictions of Inequality.* London: Routledge.

On development issues more generally:

Schaffer, B. and G. Lamb (1974) 'Exit, voice and access', *Social Science Information* **13**, pp. 73-90.

Sen, A. (1999) *Development as Freedom.* Oxford: Oxford University Press.

Sen, A. (1993) 'Capability and Well-Being', in M. Nussbaum and A. Sen (eds.) *The Quality of Life*, pp. 30-53. Oxford: Claredon.

Thomas, C. (2000) *Global Governance, Development and Human Security. The Challenge of Poverty and Inequality.* London: Pluto Press.

United Nations Development Programme (UNDP) (1990) *Human Development Report 1990.* New York: Oxford University Press.

United Nations Development Programme (UNDP) (1997) *Human Development Report 1997.* New York: Oxford University Press.

World Bank (WB) (2003) *World Development Indicators.* Washington DC: World Bank.

4. World wide web resources on HIV/AIDS mitigation in sub-Saharan Africa

The World Wide Web is an important source of information about all issues related to HIV/AIDS.[75] The first calling point for any web search on HIV/AIDS is naturally the homepage of the Joint United Nations Programme on HIV/AIDS (UNAIDS) at http://www.unaids.org. It provides among other things regularly updated epidemiological fact sheets on the state of the epidemic in each country; a bibliographical database and the possibility to download documents; and links to HIV/AIDS related activities of other international organisations.

Some of these organisations in the field of development have a special link-page for HIV/AIDS related issues, or can be searched for topical information on such issues. These include the World Bank (WB) at http://www1.worldbank.org/hiv_aids, the World Health Organisation (WHO) at http://www.who.int, the United Nations Development Programme (UNDP) at http://www.undp.org, and the United Nations Research Institute for Social Development (UNRISD) at http://www.unrisd.org.

Looking specifically at HIV/AIDS mitigation, the following web-addresses are particularly useful:

- The site of the Southern African Regional Poverty Network (SARPN) at http://www.sarpn.org.za, and here in particular the workshop report, papers and case studies from a workshop held from 27-29 May 2003 in Pretoria on 'Mitigation of HIV/AIDS Impacts through Agriculture and Rural Development - Success Stories and Future Action', all accessible through the SARPN website.
- The site of the Food and Nutrition Technical Assistance Project (FANTA) at http://www.fantaproject.org, from where a number of documents dealing with the linkages between nutrition and HIV/AIDS can be downloaded.

[75] This short guide is meant as a starting point from which special interests can then be pursued. Web-addresses were correct at the time of writing.

- The site of the African Conservation Tillage Network at http://www.act.org.zw, which promotes and facilitates sharing of information and experiences across sectors, disciplines and geographical boundaries among those involved in conservation farming practices in Africa.
- The site of the Regional Network on HIV/AIDS, Rural Livelihoods and Food Security (RENEWAL) at http://www.ifpri.org/renewal. One of the objectives of RENEWAL is to fill critical gaps in understanding how agricultural policies and programmes can contribute to prevention and/or mitigation of AIDS impact and how this knowledge can be used to support local responses. RENEWAL is currently active in Malawi, Uganda, Zambia, South Africa and Kenya.
- The site of the International AIDS Economics Network at http://www.iaen.org. From the IAEN electronic library publications dealing with, among other issues, HIV/AIDS mitigation, HIV/AIDS impact at micro and macro level, and HIV/AIDS policy issues can be downloaded.
- For a general literature search on HIV/AIDS related issues, the ELDIS Gateway to Development Information database is a useful tool, in particular the HIV/AIDS Resource Guide at http://www.eldis.org/hivaids/index.htm.

About the author

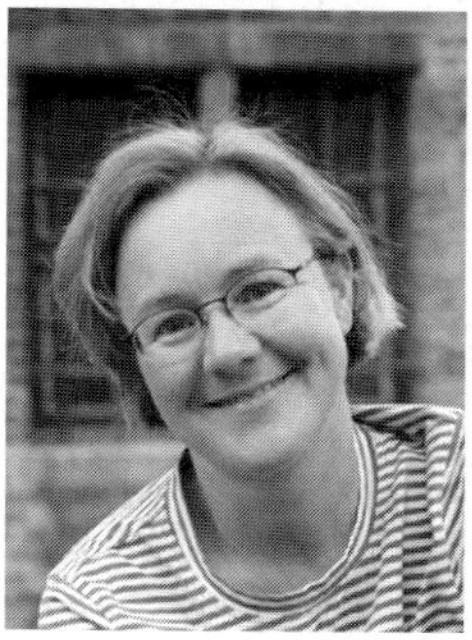

Dr. Tanja R. Müller
Department of Social Sciences
Building no. 322
Ritzema Bosweg 32A
6703 AZ Wageningen
The Netherlands
Phone: + +31-317-482038
Fax: + +31-317-482593
Email: trmdrag@yahoo.co.uk

MA in Linguistics and Philosophy (1991) at the Freie Universität Berlin; Masters in Development Studies at University College Dublin (1994); Dr. Phil in Development Studies (2003) at the University of East Anglia, Norwich, UK. Over the last ten years she has worked as: university lecturer in Dublin and Asmara; education consultant in Japan; consultant for various development projects in sub-Saharan Africa; and journalist on development issues. From June 2003 to June 2005 she was assistant professor at Wageningen University, working for the AWLAE programme mainly on the link between HIV/AIDS, food security, rural livelihoods and gender. She has published on revolution in the developing world; women, education and human resource development; African states' foreign policies; and HIV/AIDS policy issues. Her latest publication is *The Making of Elite Women. Revolution and Nation Building in Eritrea*, Boston and Leiden: Brill Publishers.

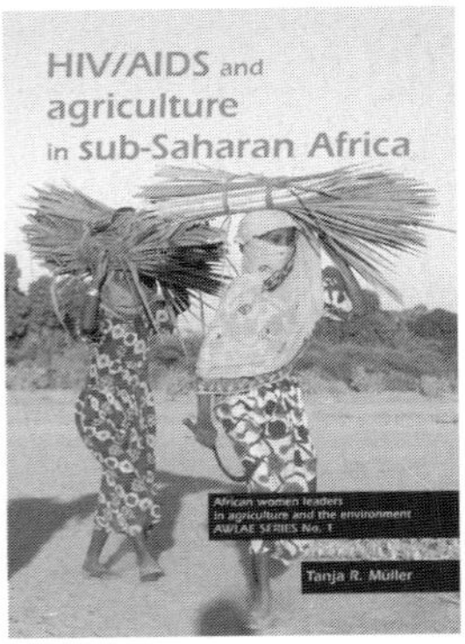

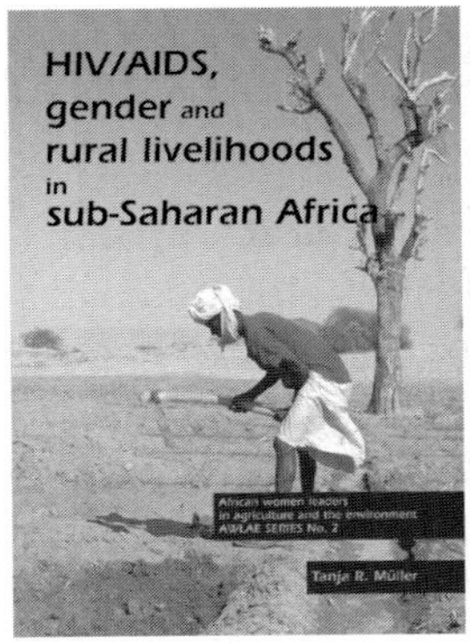

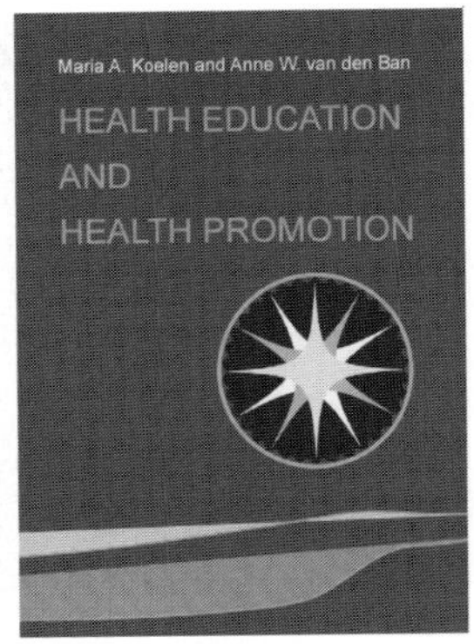

Other publications in the "African Women Leaders in Agriculture and the Environment" (AWLAE) series:

- No. 1 – HIV/AIDS and agriculture in sub-Saharan Africa: Impact on farming systems, agricultural practices and rural livelihoods An overview and annotated bibliography
  Tanja R. Müller (Wageningen University)
  ISBN: 9076998469, 2004, 104 pages, paperback, € 25

- No. 2 – HIV/AIDS, gender and rural livelihoods in sub-Saharan Africa An overview and annotated bibliography
  Tanja R. Müller (Wageningen University)
  ISBN: 9076998493, 2005, 120 pages, paperback, € 25

Other publications from Wageningen Academic Publishers:

- Health education and health promotion
  Maria A. Koelen and Anne W. van den Ban
  ISBN: 9076998442, 2004, 288 pages, paperback, € 45

These publications are available at:
Wageningen Academic Publishers
P.O. Box 220
6700 AE Wageningen
The Netherlands
sales@WageningenAcademic.com
www.WageningenAcademic.com